Aviation Psychology:
Applied Methods and Techniques

Ioana V. Koglbauer and
Sonja Biede-Straussberger
(Eds.)

Aviation Psychology

Applied Methods and Techniques

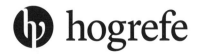 hogrefe

Library of Congress Cataloging in Publication information for the print version of this book is available via the Library of Congress Marc Database under the LC Control Number 2021937702

Library and Archives Canada Cataloguing in Publication
Title: Aviation psychology : applied methods and techniques / Ioana V. Koglbauer and
Sonja Biede-Straussberger (eds.).
Other titles: Aviation psychology (2021)
Names: Koglbauer, Ioana V., editor. | Biede-Straussberger, Sonja, editor.
Description: Includes bibliographical references.
Identifiers: Canadiana (print) 20210205326 | Canadiana (ebook) 20210205377 | ISBN 9780889375888
(softcover) | ISBN 9781616765880 (PDF) | ISBN 9781613345887 (EPUB)
Subjects: LCSH: Aviation psychology.
Classification: LCC RC1085 .A95 2021 | DDC 155.9/65—dc23

© 2021 by Hogrefe Publishing
www.hogrefe.com

PUBLISHING OFFICES
USA: Hogrefe Publishing Corporation, 361 Newbury Street, 5th Floor, Boston, MA 02115
                Phone (857) 880-2002; E-mail customerservice@hogrefe.com
EUROPE: Hogrefe Publishing GmbH, Merkelstr. 3, 37085 Göttingen, Germany
                Phone +49 551 99950-0, Fax +49 551 99950-111; E-mail publishing@hogrefe.com
SALES & DISTRIBUTION
USA: Hogrefe Publishing, Customer Services Department,
                30 Amberwood Parkway, Ashland, OH 44805
                Phone (800) 228-3749, Fax (419) 281-6883; E-mail customerservice@hogrefe.com
UK: Hogrefe Publishing, c/o Marston Book Services Ltd., 160 Eastern Ave., Milton Park,
                Abingdon, OX14 4SB
                Phone +44 1235 465577, Fax +44 1235 465556; E-mail direct.orders@marston.co.uk
EUROPE: Hogrefe Publishing, Merkelstr. 3, 37085 Göttingen, Germany
                Phone +49 551 99950-0, Fax +49 551 99950-111; E-mail publishing@hogrefe.com
OTHER OFFICES
CANADA: Hogrefe Publishing, 82 Laird Drive, East York, Ontario, M4G 3V1
SWITZERLAND: Hogrefe Publishing, Länggass-Strasse 76, 3012 Bern

Printed and bound in Germany

ISBN 978-0-88937-588-8 (print) · ISBN 978-1-61676-588-0 (PDF) · ISBN 978-1-61334-588-7 (EPUB)
https://doi.org/10.1027/00588-000

Dedication

The editors and contributing authors dedicate this book to Professor K. Wolfgang Kallus. Over several decades, Wolfgang's contributions have benchmarked the theoretical and methodological foundation for advancements in the research and application of aviation psychology. Among the contributions we would like to highlight: dedicated teaching at the University of Graz; creating and organizing the International Summer School on Aviation Psychology (ISAP) from 2003 to 2019; conducting research projects with EUROCONTROL, Austro Control GmbH, and the aviation industry. At a time when many psychologists focused their research on isolated phenomena, Wolfgang fostered an interdisciplinary approach and brought together in his projects a diverse bunch of experts such as psychologists, psychophysiologists, engineers, pilots, air traffic controllers, and medical experts. With the International Summer School on Aviation Psychology, Wolfgang gathered together renowned international experts who gave presentations and workshops to a mixed audience consisting of psychologists, students, and people involved in aviation operations. Wolfgang fostered professional excellence, interdisciplinarity, and connectivity that are core values of the aviation psychology community and of the European Association for Aviation Psychology (EAAP). In 2012 Wolfgang was presented with the EAAP Award for his outstanding international commitment and achievement in aviation psychology and human factors. Many chapters of this volume address areas that have been advanced by the contributions of Wolfgang, his students, and his collaborators. Wolfgang valued a multidimensional approach for accessing information and consequently for understanding human behavior. He addressed the individual and organizational perspective in order to highlight how individual behavior and performance are influenced by the organization. Furthermore, he investigated in parallel subjective and objective data, including psychophysiological measures. Wolfgang approached the dynamics of human behavior with particular interest in stress and recovery. He valued the integrative and interdisciplinary ways of working, created and facilitated international research networks, and inspired new generations of aviation psychologists. While the editors aimed to create a volume on current topics in aviation psychology, this book also honors Professor K. Wolfgang Kallus.

Acknowledgments

The editors would like to thank Michaela Schwarz, President of the European Association for Aviation Psychology (EAAP), and the Board of Directors of the EAAP – Gunnar Steinhardt, Renée Pelchen-Medwed, Karina Mesarosova, Mickaël Causse, Jennifer Eaglestone, and Robert Bor – for supporting this book project. Each chapter in this book was reviewed by two independent peer reviewers. We thank the reviewers who conducted peer reviews of the chapters. We gratefully acknowledge the former EAAP Presidents Peter Jorna and André Droog for their valuable feedback. In addition, the editors thankfully acknowledge the dedicated team at Hogrefe Publishing – from commissioning to publishing and marketing – for their assistance.

Contents

Foreword

Peter Jorna

Human Factor(s): What Do You Do With It?

That was the title of my first colloquium presentation at the Netherlands Aerospace Laboratory (NLR) around 1990. The audience at that time was made up of all kinds of engineers, some scientists, and a couple of engineering pilots. All of them wondering why all these wonderful aircraft were crashing due to pilot error. Workload was apparently an issue and several attempts had already been made to model the human mathematically as a biological part of the aircraft control loop. But pilots did not recognize themselves or their personalities in the description of a variable amplification factor in complex equations that were meant to simulate the effects of their workload. This approach was not accepted as being very useful. It faded away ...

The presentation explained that humans as test subjects (now called "participants") are indeed an important part of the control loops, but that the test procedures that had been used to date were either not including the human as a to-be-tested part of the system at all or the tests were way too crude to have any predictive value. Test pilots were the main representatives of flight crew, but they were exceptionally well trained. Thus, they did not really represent "the minimum pilot" who sometimes has to perform under harsh working conditions, being tired, distracted, recently divorced etc. A different, more system- and context-oriented testing perspective was needed.

Some steps were taken over the following years.

Go Beyond Selection

The Royal Netherlands Navy at that time had an issue with pilots who were able to fly the new maritime patrol aircraft but had problems when combining the flying with fighting. Hunting submarines at low altitude above the sea was not only exciting and risky, but also required the use of an additional computer screen on the flight deck showing tactical information and instructions, creating a "dual-task situation" in psychology language. Some licensed pilots could not do that and were not able to obtain operational status.

The management response in those days was (most often) to seek the problem in the humans (blame culture), and thus improved selection was the way to go. Selection research following navy trainees during their career confirmed there were individual differences in the capability of (male) pilots to do two things at the same time (either parallel or by fast serial task switching), but training was also an important factor. The aviation industry had no idea about the existence and relevance of individual differences between users of new technologies: An illustration of the fact that simply adding a display aimed at improving mission performance by presenting extra data to the pilot is not an instant guarantee that it will pay off for everybody. On the contrary, the licensed pilots who could not become operational were now a major cost factor for the navy.

Perhaps better test and validation should be recommended already during the design stage?

Go Beyond Subjective Opinion(s)

Asking for user opinions is an easy and very tempting method to check your design. But do the users understand the new design? Are they in favor of it or afraid that it will change their jobs? The EUROCONTROL PHARE program (Programme for Harmonised Air Traffic Management [ATM] Research in Europe) included my so-called ground human machine interface (GHMI) project. In this project several human factors specialists and psychologists teamed up to develop a detailed specification of the human–machine interface for future ATM. There was no explaining to others how to do it, but just do it by ourselves. That task allocation was a really good idea made by Mick van Gool who was the PHARE program manager at the time. Part of this project allowed for some experimental research. The big discussion at that time was whether automation in the form of computer advice to the controller would be a help or a burden.

The reasoning was as follows. If the controller would compare the advice with their own idea, it would involve an extra task, thus a burden. In the case of high task/traffic load, the task of comparing advice with one's own idea could be simply dropped, meaning that the advice of a software tool would be ignored. Alternatively, one could simply follow the advice under high individual workload conditions, but in that case the controller would be "out of the loop." A clear dilemma to be solved.

A simulation study at NLR by Brian Hilburn made a comparison between controllers working with various levels of automation support and the "normal" manual control mode. The results revealed clear and consistent workload benefits as a function of the level of automation and in comparison with manual control as a reference. Benefits were reflected in physiological measures (e.g., heart rate, heart rate variability, pupil size) indicating both lower mental effort or stress and better performance (response times to da-talink communication). All these measures indicated the positive effects of automation, and thus less burden and not more. Except for one other meas-urement: the subjective ratings of workload by the controllers. This meas-ure was the only indicator that went up. A big surprise and a clear dissocia-tion between measures.

Closer analysis and friendly discussions with controllers revealed that their cognitive reasoning was, "I have to do my normal work and deal with additional tools," so "more tools must mean more work." This lesson learned about possible dissociations between measurements has been experienced more often in research on workload, and therefore it is always necessary and mandatory to measure performance, mental effort, and subjective ap-preciation in concert. Know your methods and how to apply them!

Validate With Humans in the Loop

These experiences showed us that all technical claims assuming better human performance or reduced workload by adding some technology need to be validated and proven. Merely adding colors to a computer screen does not justify the claim that colors will decrease workload. Evidence is always better. Asking pilots and air traffic controllers will provide you with valua-ble and interesting opinions, but beside the reliability or validity issue there is the popular saying: "Ask 10 pilots and you will get 20 different opinions." Who has the right opinion? This is a necessary and informative method, but not sufficient.

Take Objective Measures Related to the Human Task

Making a detailed (and agreed upon) task description is the starting point, as it already helps to reduce misinterpretations between the various disci-plines involved. Also measures for various task performance aspects should be defined as objectively as possible; for example, in terms of time, the qual-ity of human performance and its measurable influence on system param-eters. Task definition (what is allocated to the human) is a good starting point, but is only completed if you can define measurements. When is a task performed better, and how can I detect and measure this? Note that task considerations are now also integrated in the airworthiness regulations of aircraft. Rule 25.1302 addresses the certification of "installed systems for use by the flight crew" and it requires a task-based perspective for defining the system challenges in terms of information required, controls needed, and automation support that is understandable and predictable for the users. A real human factors regulation.

But it is even better to also have an idea or hypothesis about the estimated and actual level of effort, especially mental effort, because good performance should be maintainable for a full mission or working period. In this respect, psychophysiological methods came to the rescue. Heart rate and heart rate variability (HRV) provided indications of both physical as well as mental aspects of work, including emotions.

Hard data always work better, also in certification to convince people, including managers and agencies.

Accept the Help of Our Psychophysiology Friends

My first great helper in getting psychophysiology accepted was Glenn Wilson from the Wright Patterson Air Force Base in the United States. He managed to get some heart rate data measured from pilots in real jet aircraft flying missions as well as in the simulators. Not easy to obtain.

What a difference in response between real flying and simulation! The data clearly revealed the limits in simulator realism. Pilots know that simulators do not kill.

My second great helper was Wolfgang Kallus, a German gentleman who got lost in Austria in the wonderful and beautiful town of Graz. He used psychophysiology in an impressive way and was also involved in the ongoing mission to convince people that aviation psychology is absolutely relevant and necessary for design, operational performance, and safety. Find the problems with human–machine interaction before the accidents!

Do not Just Criticize, but Educate

Wolfgang quickly realized that education is a key factor for progress in the field of aviation psychology and human factors in its application and integration in aviation. There are excellent psychologists who know a lot about the human brain and behavior, but many are ignorant about flying machines or air traffic control decisions. No one in aviation will take them seriously if they do not speak "the language." So, the psychologists need to be educated about systems and operations in order to become *aviation psychologists*.

Similarly, there are pilots, controllers, maintainance technicians etc. who all have a great interest in the fascinating human factors of their own work area but lack detailed education about psychology, let alone understand its methodologies. Wolfgang and his excellent team brought such people with all their different backgrounds together in Graz. And it worked! Wolfgang was the first to organize an International Summer School on Aviation Psychology (ISAP) that provided dedicated familiarization, education, sharing, and training in aviation psychology. For everybody.

Wolfgang and his highly appreciated teams were awarded the special trophy of the European Association for Aviation Psychology (EAAP) for their contributions to aviation psychology and its applications in human factors.

Now There Is a Book on *How to Do It!*

The ISAP and EAAP work together in sharing information and experience, but Wolfgang went a little further. He did his very best to refine and expand all kinds of methods and procedures to improve the impact (a bad word to use in the aviation context, but a reminder of why we do this ...) of aviation psychology on the safety, well-being, and performance of all humans working in or using aviation.

Many collaborators, former students, and friends of Wolfgang contributed to this volume. This book presents some of the recent lessons learned in applying aviation psychology and human factors, and what methods work best for what purpose.

We hope that the tradition of ISAP will continue and that the book may have regular updates in the future. Use the book as a source and inspiration for others in the future.

Now the task we all have for the continuation of what has been accomplished: Tell and help others!

Professor Peter Jorna
In tribute to Professor Wolfgang Kallus
Friends and allies in the "battle" for human factors integration

Preface

Sonja Biede-Straussberger and Ioana V. Koglbauer

The idea for this book arose from a discussion of the current status of aviation psychology at a professional meeting with key European players involved in professional domains such as universities, institutes, and the European Association for Aviation Psychology (EAAP). This meeting took place in Toulouse, one of the European bases of aviation. Toulouse is an exciting place, connecting major aviation contributors, such as a worldwide leading aircraft manufacturer and related industries, a civil aviation organization, along with schools providing operational and professional education for this sector.

Aviation is a field that connects people and countries, to exchange and to explore, and as such it is not surprising that the people participating in this meeting were former students of Wolfgang Kallus, who, as psychologists, pondered ideas to reinforce the role of aviation psychology and human factors in the industry. One of these questions addressed the ways of working that professionals in the field use to make sure that a full integration of aviation psychology is no longer a wish but a reality across the aeronautical system. A way to support this is by sharing knowledge and experience, and thus the idea for the topic of this book was born.

Practical application of aviation psychology covers the design and assessment of various areas such as human roles, human–machine systems, procedures, airspaces, and airports. It requires an interdisciplinary approach from their initial design through to operational deployment. However, published research in aviation psychology reflects only a small part of the actual work done. A large part of research and development is conducted behind closed doors in the industry. Results of cooperations between industry and academia are not published for various reasons, among which are questions of competitiveness, security, or simply the time available to share lessons learnt.

But what are the enablers of successful applications of aviation psychology? Several may be listed, starting by ensuring the diversity of competencies that professionals require to flexibly adapt to the continuously evolving requirements of the aeronautical landscape. Other enablers include establishing efficient support to newcomers, or the regular evolution of learning curricula while taking on board the evolution of society. One of these enablers is sharing comprehensive views on key topics and lessons learnt regarding approaches, methods, and tools.

Hence, the objective of this book is to provide the reader with a selection of views and practices highly relevant in aviation psychology. Aviation psychology is about the application of scientific knowledge on human behavior to the various areas of aviation, ranging from research, design, to operation. The human is a complex system with plenty of limitations and opportunities to fail due to their inherent characteristics, but the human is also a creative and adaptive system. As such it is the leading element that can intervene and rescue a situation when things go wrong, that is able to innovate and improve, and that is dynamic and flexible to manage the variability of the working environment. One of these situations occurred when Kevin Sullivan experienced unexpected aircraft behavior in Qantas Flight 72. The pilot shares this experience in his book *No Man's Land*. The crew successfully landed the aircraft and hence saved the lives of the passengers on board thanks to the strengths of the humans in that situation. But more than that, it describes the role of psychology, as it relates the strong interplay between human and machine, but also between all the people and organizations involved, and the strong association between the time before and after the event. Another example of the unique capability of human performance was given by the air traffic controller Lou Ella Hollingsworth, who saved a crew's life in November 2012. She detected the incapacitation of the pilot flying a Piaggio P180 Avanti at high altitude because his speech on the frequency was slurred and incoherent. She thought the crew was suffering from hypoxia, as also suggested by another pilot who heard the communication on the frequency. Calmly and firmly, Lou Ella repeatedly advised the pilot to descend and put on his oxygen mask, thus finding a solution that was beyond typical air traffic control procedures. The pilot put on the oxygen mask, descended, recovered, and safely continued his flight. These and many other examples show that the human is the core element of the aviation system and, thus, human performance deserves special attention.

In the context of continuous changes in society and technology that impact aviation to a large extent, a deeper integration of the knowledge of psychology in organizations and in technical developments is essential. At the same time, taking a central view of the role of the human is necessary so as to meet the future expectations regarding the operational performance of the aeronautical system as a whole while ensuring human wellbeing and performance. Over the past few decades, the knowledge base of psychology has continued to grow, as it has in neighboring disciplines of psychology. Today, psychology can be seen as being increasingly diffused over the different areas of society, including aviation. Today, we also have more knowledge of neurosciences, anthropometrics, sociology, and anthropology, and of how phenomena are connected thanks to largely available and promoted data sharing.

As such, it is a major challenge for any of us professionals to choose the appropriate knowledge to guarantee that the human element is receiving the right level of attention in the field. To make sure that we are doing aviation psychology right, we need to ensure that we effectively and efficiently use the experience and knowledge available. In the Foreword of this book, Peter Jorna described the learning of an organization over time with regard to how the view on human factors evolved and became increasingly integrated to solve actual problems. Today we have the opportunity to understand how such learning occurred in the past. But we also have the opportunity to go one step further, by bringing together the knowledge that exists, what we have learnt, and how to connect it to anticipate the future. The challenge is to make sure we can share the lessons learnt. We want to avoid that future generations of professionals in the evolving fields of aviation experience the same situations as Peter reported in the Foreword. Especially in the context of increasing economic pressure and changing ways of working, human tendencies for regression and repeating the same story as already experienced in the past could prevail.

Thus, we want to use this opportunity to report on the experiences learnt in the past, to share knowledge that was gathered, and to build on the lessons learnt. The authors of this book work in the industry, in research institutions, public services or operations. They share their experiences with the application of different methods, some difficulties encountered, and an outlook ahead. Therefore, this toolkit of aviation psychology provides the reader with know-how that is otherwise not easy to access.

Over the past few decades, the knowledge base on aviation psychology has also evolved in international standardization and regulation that set a global framework for professionals in the field. For example, for more than a decade, aircraft certification has required a human factors demonstration, and the role of aviation psychologists has been emphasized in a new rule on support. However, aviation psychologists need to assess, to select, and sometimes to develop new methods for addressing practical and theoretical challenges in their work. This book provides an overview of current themes, methods, and tools, and offers complementary views on topics presented in journals. These are selected to cover academic and industrial areas of interest, and have different foci such as psychophysiology, people in organizations, and design processes.

This book starts with an introduction of the Human Performance Assessment Process, which is now widely used in aviation ranging from assessment of aircraft to air traffic control. This process was developed to a large extent in SESAR 1, the first step of the European Single Sky Aviation Research Program between 2010 and 2016, and is currently the baseline for ensuring the study of human performance even beyond SESAR. What is essential here is that the authors involved in this activity, together with many other experts, built on their own past experience to reinforce the integration of human factors in the industry and in operations. As such the authors not only connect countries (Austria, Germany, Italy, France), but also cover different organizations (from research to operations, from aircraft manufacturers to air traffic management). They overcame the challenge of remaining stuck in their own organizational constraints, and devoted themselves to building together for a common future based on the lessons they learnt. Everyone who wants to mitigate human performance issues – including automation issues – in the design phase of a concept and beyond, towards deployment, may find interest in reading this chapter. The chapter raises awareness of existing challenges and provides guidance on how to optimize human performance integration in system design. Together with the second chapter, it shows how aviation psychology builds bridges across disciplines and application fields. It takes two perspectives, first by integrating aviation psychology in engineering and design processes across multiple connected organizations and products, but also by bridging the gap between research and applications. In this context, professionals are also given the opportunity to choose the right methods and tools according to the available constraints. A dedicated chapter on bridging gaps highlights that the currently available criteria for selecting methods and tools are no longer sufficient, as we need to take a global system-of-systems perspective to identify the areas in which problems have to be addressed. For this purpose, the human-oriented approach of interactions with complexity (HOAC) is presented. One of the challenges the authors have encountered is to develop the right set of human factor criteria in an industrial context and make sure it is used throughout the design process. Keeping a system-of-systems perspective was always a key driver in their reflections.

A special chapter is dedicated to an organization-focused view regarding "Essential Tools for Safety Culture Development in Air Traffic Management." Safety culture is a current topic in aviation psychology that is being regularly assessed and interpreted in aviation operations (e.g., air navigation services). The authors of this chapter have experience in airline and air traffic control operations, and share practical tips and tricks for a reliable, cost- and time-efficient application. This chapter raises awareness about scientifically validated tools for assessing, monitoring, and improving safety culture in aviation organizations. It provides an opportunity to learn how to successfully apply these tools in the operational context and how to make results tangible for operational staff. It also explains the derivation of meaningful results and interpretations of safety culture assessments.

Specific cognitive processes and the relationships to physiology are highlighted in the chapters on anticipation and spatial disorientation. One chapter is dedicated to anticipative processes both in flying an aircraft and in air traffic control. Pilots and controllers are expected to be "ahead" of a situation. What are the processes that enable them to see a situation developing in the way they want it to, instead of being surprised and reacting to a multitude of constantly changing elements? How can estimations of collisions be effectively improved to achieve an accuracy of a fraction of a second? How are anticipative processes reflected in human psychophysiology? This chapter presents theoretical and practical hands-on applications and answers these questions on anticipative processes. In addition, the reader will discover tools and examples for designing aviation systems that assist human operators in their anticipative processing. A promising outlook at new developments of anticipatory processes for artificial intelligence is deemed to inspire the next generation of researchers and practitioners in aviation psychology.

Another chapter on cognition is written by an expert in spatial disorientation research. This chapter serves as a practical guide through various research methods, applicable to the field of spatial disorientation. It describes examples of studies from the literature, with an emphasis on research methodologies. Furthermore, it contributes to a better understanding of how spatial disorientation can impact pilot performance and flight safety.

Several chapters are dedicated to a deeper reflection on psychophysiology in aviation. The chapter on reactivity addresses a basic biophysiological paradigm. An understanding of reactivity is essential for predicting human performance and error management in high-reliability environments such as aviation. Reactivity concepts contribute to elucidating individuals' reactions in social settings and, thus, to better prediction of behavior and performance. Key methodological aspects for addressing reactivity are presented and explained from a joint perspective: medicine, psychology, and work safety.

Another key concept in understanding human performance is described in the chapter on stress recovery. The importance of stress management for safe human performance is recognized and addressed by the European Commission and by the European Union Aviation Safety Agency (EASA) in recent regulations, guidelines, and standards for pilots and air traffic controllers (e.g., peer support, critical incident stress management, stress management education). This chapter on psychophysiological regeneration is particularly interesting for understanding, predicting, and managing human performance in the dynamic and safety-critical aviation domain.

Finally, experience in the application of psychophysiological measures is shared by taking a specific focus on the use of cardiac and electrodermal activity assessment as well as eye-tracking methods in aviation. A special chapter is dedicated to eye-tracking methods used to analyze pilots' activity beyond the laboratory, in ecological settings. For several years, the authors have been dedicated to finding solutions for efficiently integrating objective measures on human behavior in an industrial environment. This chapter explains specific methods for conducting an eye-tracking study in the cockpit, such as determining the sample frequency and the algorithms for detecting fixations and saccades. In addition, the chapter explains how eye-tracking parameters can be used to test research hypotheses related to pilot behavior and local areas of interest in the cockpit. Furthermore, the synchronization of an eye-tracker with other physiological sensors is explained for a more comprehensive assessment of human performance in the cockpit.

The chapter on applications of cardiac and electrodermal activity assessment in aviation shows what can be achieved when a psychologist and an engineer, who are also enthusiastic pilots, put their heads together to conquer a cross-domain problem. This chapter addresses aspects such as the reliability and sensitivity of cardiac and electrodermal parameters in real flight with high acceleration and in spaceflight in conditions of microgravity. The chapter describes methods and results of cardiac and electrodermal data collection and analysis, as well as lessons learnt from various aviation studies. Furthermore, the authors show how applications of cardiac and electrodermal parameters can be used to advance the assessment of pilot training and for the design of biocybernetics systems (e.g., adaptive automation).

The users of aviation psychology knowledge are very diverse, ranging from psychologists and human factors specialists to operational experts, trainers, etc. What is essential is to share a global understanding within this diverse user community. One is often stuck in one's own work, but opening up to different ideas and approaches can bring benefits that one has not considered before. Even though the knowledge shared in this book may be perceived as applicable only to aviation, it can be used for global awareness and open exchanges across domains.

Now it is time to look towards the future. A lot of our experience as professionals in the field of aviation psychology is based on ways of working that were determined by the key drivers of society in the past decade. They may no longer be the determining ones for the future. Our society is currently undergoing a major transformation due to technical developments but also socioeconomic changes. Digitalization, distributed work places, or different expectations that people have towards employers continue to set the stage for reflecting on future needs. This will also impact our methods and tools, which will have to evolve even more to adapt better, used to study and demonstrate that future procedures and systems will be aligned with the principles of human performance capability. However, we as a professional community have our current experience to build upon. It will allow us to examine how to anticipate and prepare faster to meet future needs, to develop methods and tools for this future context, and to be ready to embrace future challenges. A real target for aviation psychologists is to be proactive and to remain ahead. We also need to be engaged in the design and assessment of aviation systems. Thus, the work of an aviation psychologist is more efficient in the prevention than in the investigation of accidents and incidents. In the past, aviation psychologists were mainly asked to explain what went wrong, as Peter Jorna vividly illustrated in the Foreword of this volume. Our aim is to be involved in all phases of system design and operations. Thus, aviation psychologists with the right knowledge and tools can predict human performance and can contribute to a better and safer human performance integration.

Chapter 1

The Evolution Toward a Common Air/Ground Framework for Human Performance Assessments in Europe

Renée Pelchen-Medwed, Luca Save, Alexander Heintz, Florence Reuzeau, and Sonja Biede-Straussberger

Abstract

This chapter describes the evolution of approaches and methods for human factors (HF) integration in design and implementation across air traffic management (ATM), encompassing industry, operations, and regulations. To outline recent methods in the European system engineering and performance framework, the SESAR Human Performance Assessment Process, the SESAR Level of Automation Taxonomy (LOAT) and their evolution are described in detail. Major achievements such as the integration of air and ground roles and perspectives widening the scope from design to transition factors, including training, staffing, social factors, and change management, as well as a more integrated understanding of the human role in the entire aviation system are addressed. Ongoing challenges and lessons learnt, for example, concerning availability and interdisciplinarity of HF competence, integration of air/ ground issues, or links to performance and safety-related assessments are discussed.

Keywords: air traffic management, digitalization, big data, artificial intelligence, automation, human performance

Introduction

The role of human factors (HF) in the design, development, evaluation, and implementation of air traffic management (ATM) systems is critical as only a perfectly integrated system in the widest sense will ensure the required performance. Human operators should be considered at a large scale. These are pilots, cabin crew, airport and air traffic control staff, instructors, maintenance personnel, and many more. Among the performance principles to be noted are safety; operational and customer efficiency; health, wellbeing, and safety for the human operators; compliance with regulations; and differentiation opportunities against the competition. The development of HF engineering approaches is directly linked to the expected benefits and performance requirements. Multifaceted HF issues can be a result of the inappropriate design of large human–machine systems. In this case the system design does not consider sufficiently the requirements and needs of the human operators. Today, the community has found and implemented approaches to ensure these issues are managed. This was, however, not as obvious when the first initiatives preparing the future ATM system were started.

History of the Human Factors Integration Process

During the 1990s, the Programme for Harmonised ATM Research in EUROCONTROL (PHARE) was initiated involving a number of European research institutions. By sharing Air Traffic Control (ATC) and aeronautics experience, the goal was to study the future air–ground integrated ATM system in all flight phases making use of precise four-dimensional trajectories in an air/ground datalink environment.

Even though the basic principles of today's ATM programs were set at this time, HF had not yet started to be systematically integrated within such a large program. First initiatives were explored to integrate HF as part of a multidisciplinary team in human–machine interface (HMI) specifications. And already at this time it was noted, "...that HF work was largely underdone within academic circles, whereas ATC system development was an industrial exercise" (EUROCONTROL, 1999, p. 21). At that time the recommendation stated that, "human factors within PHARE should be organized as a single coherent program so that findings from each part can be interpreted in relation to the whole, and not take the form of a series of unconnected items" (EUROCONTROL, 1999, p. 21).

In parallel, EUROCONTROL launched the Human Factors and Manpower Unit, which addressed HF integration in future ATM systems (HIFA). Within this unit, the so-called HF case (EUROCONTROL, 2007) was developed to systematically manage the identification and treatment of HF issues as early as possible in a project life cycle. European partners continued, for example, in the project Episode 3, to clarify and detail the role of the HF case and how it is associated with other perspectives of the performance assessment of ATM concepts, such as the safety case, business case, or other.

Starting from a wider reach of the academic impact of HF, from the late 1990s on, air navigation service providers (ANSPs) started integrating HF specialists within their organizations. Organizations such as NATS, DFS, Skyguide, Frequentis, ENAV, or Thales have set up HF groups that were and often still are mostly allocated within research domains. Consequently, the way that HF specialists were involved in system design varied, and HF specialists were hardly ever involved along the complete validation and verification cycle of a project.

At the same time, HF as a systematic discipline also emerged in the airborne domain. In Aerospatiale manufacturing (previous Airbus company), the first ergonomics department was set up in 1984. The development of *work analysis* methodology and *ergonomics referential* made it possible to support the introduction of new machines and tools in the product lines. Job instruction and training definition were outlined and maintained by the ergonomists. Since 1993, each plant and final assembly lines have retained the services of an ergonomist. They pooled their effort in a network animated by an ergonomist coordinator.

In the early 1990s, HF organizations were formally integrated in the design offices. The first Airbus technical note related to the integration of HF in the system engineering process was issued in 1999. During the ensuing years, aviation manufacturers, suppliers, researchers, and regulators have developed a qualitative approach in HF up to defining a new basis for HF regulations in 2004: the CS 25-1302 (European Aviation Safety Agency, EASA, 2007), and then the AC 25-1302 (Federal Aviation Administration, FAA, 2013). This can be interpreted as a certain level of maturity in HF knowledge applied to aviation. Today, an HF design process is fully described and embedded in the main processes of the company by addressing the human performance and limitations (HPL) of all operators working on products, services, and processes (aircraft, training, documentation etc.; Reuzeau, 2019).

Next to various local European initiatives to establish HF expertise, HF groups developed worldwide. The HF groups of FAA and NASA established a number of support activities that are shared with the worldwide community, such as the FAA Human Factors Design Standard (HFDS; Ahlstrom & Longo, 2003).

Additionally, standards such as ISO 9241 that provide guidance on how to consider HF during a design phase were developed. Besides, there are international norms used in other domains such as the military. The UK Ministry of Defence (MOD) has defined standards on HF integration (Ministry of Defence, 2015), and processes also exist for the nuclear domain and railway. However, the amount and way of their application still vary.

How Did It Start? The Early Stages of the SESAR Human Performance Assessment Process

Despite all these developments, the foundation of the largest European ATM R&D program SESAR (originally SESAME) based on an initiative of the aircraft and system manufacturer industry required a new set-up to establish systematic integration of HF into development and implementation of new and increasingly automated systems (Heintz & Merz, 2012). As the majority of the proposed operational improvements within SESAR were related to automation in various areas and technical improvements in the ATM/CNS domain, the effects on the core resource to provide ATM, namely, the human actors, were still not addressed systematically, notwithstanding the complex interaction of the various elements of the "system" aviation in the widest sense. To achieve a holistic view of the entire aviation system, the classic areas of system design, training, selection, social factors, and change management were subsumed under the term "human performance." During SESAR's definition phase the focus was on an interdisciplinary high-level impact assessment for these three areas (i.e., automation principles, estimation of training effort, and impacts on staffing and work relations) and on complementing the operational concept as well as the "European ATM Master Plan" from a human performance perspective (e.g., SESAR, 2007a, 2007b, 2009). Consequently, the succeeding SESAR development phase under the SESAR joint undertaking (European Commission, EUROCONTROL, and various industry partners from the entire European aviation industry) led to the development of a framework to systematically integrate all aspects of human performance (HP), the Human Performance Assessment Process (HPAP; SESAR Joint Undertaking, 2016). Today, many years after the integration of HF in organizations was initiated, the Single European Sky ATM Research (SESAR) program allows for real cooperation between partners across different industries.

The SESAR Human Performance Assessment Process (HPAP)

Once the need for a new HF integration process for SESAR was clearly identified, requirements for the process development were formulated.

As Chalon-Morgan et al. (2012) describe, these are:

1. A consistent approach to HF integration for operational and technical projects; and

2. The possibility to aggregate HF impacts and associate them with the ATM target performance criteria.

Consequently, between 2010 and 2014 a systematic HPAP was developed to meet these requirements. The methodology for SESAR is based on existing HF integration processes used across the aviation industry. One example of such a process is the EUROCONTROL HF Case (EUROCONTROL, 2007).

The HPAP accompanies an operational concept from the design phase to the development phase. The aim is to prevent and mitigate potential negative impacts that are caused by inadequate consideration of human capabilities and limitations. A systematic identification of recommendations and/or requirements ensures that a design corresponds to the human needs.

The skeleton of the HP assessment process comprises the following four steps (Chalon-Morgan et al., 2012): Step 1, understand the ATM concept; Step 2, understand HP implications; Step 3, improve and validate the concept; and Step 4, collate findings and produce the HP assessment report.

The HPAP adopted a systematic argument and evidence-based approach in line with different safety methodologies.

As the authors further detailed (Chalon-Morgan et al., 2012):

A human performance argument can be understood in this context as "a human performance claim that has to be proven." The HP arguments are structured into four different HF areas, namely:

1. Human roles;
2. Human and the system;
3. Teams and communication; and
4. Transition factors (which includes general acceptability, training, skills and competencies, and staffing). (p. 248)

Each of the four main high-level arguments is broken down into lower-level, more detailed arguments to be able to identify HP issues. For example, Argument 1 – the role of the human is consistent with human capabilities and limitations – is subdivided into: "Argument 1.1, Roles and responsibilities of human actors are clear and exhaustive; Argument 1.2, Operating methods are clear and support human performance; and Argument 1.3, Human actors can achieve their tasks (under normal, abnormal, and degraded modes of operations." In turn, Argument 1.1 is further broken down into: "1.1.1, The description of roles and responsibilities covers all affected human actors"; and "1.1.2, The description of roles and responsibilities covers all tasks to be performed by a human operator" and so forth. (p. 248)

For each argument, the evidence required to satisfy the specific argument is defined. Each argument is linked to a set of suggested HP activities to ensure that the consideration of HP implications is not merely stated or taken for granted. Systematically covering all arguments prevents missing critical aspects that influence overall system performance and, in turn, a successful and timely implementation.

Following the initial description in the work of Biede-Straussberger and Pelchen-Medwed (2017), the following section recalls the essential characteristics of each step, as referred to by the authors.

In Step 1, an understanding of the ATM concept is acquired by reviewing relevant project documentations and in-depth discussions with the concept developers to determine the change between the reference and the solution concept. HP-related assumptions are defined and agreed and the HP level of maturity is determined using the maturity criteria provided in the HP reference material (SESAR, 2016).

In Step 2, after identifying the relevant high-level HP arguments, the HP argument structure is used to filter the relevant lower-level arguments. Once the low-level arguments are known, the HF expert can identify the related HP issues with the help of operational specialists. "The issues and benefits are described in terms of their impact on human and system performance and rated in terms. Where possible, actions to address or mitigate the issue are identified." (Biede-Straussberger & Pelchen-Medwed, 2017, p. 3).

Once the arguments are identified, the guidance material points the project team toward the required HP activity(ies) (e.g., workshops, task analyses, real-time simulations) and the associated evidence. This results in an initial HP assessment plan. Further on, the refinement and prioritization of HP activities, HP issues, and benefits will be reviewed by considering previous literature, related concepts, and stakeholder inputs.

The HP assessment plan describes each HP activity. This activity description consists of the following elements:

> The arguments and issues to be addressed and hence the HP objectives of the activity; the required evidence (or success criteria); and the general planning of the activity, i.e., timeline, resource and approach, so that they can be understood and discussed with the project manager and project team members including the safety and validation teams. The HP assessment plan is a key element to be integrated in the project's validation plan. (Biede-Straussberger & Pelchen-Medwed, 2017, p. 3)

Step 3 covers the major effort required to conduct the HP activities. The data collected have to be analyzed and documented. The results not only represent evidence, but also lead to recommendations and requirements. These have to be discussed, consolidated, and prioritized with the other members of the project team.

Step 4 assesses whether sufficient evidence has been gathered, whether the concept can proceed to the next maturity step, and, finally, the HP assessment report is developed.

The SESAR eHP repository (https://ext.eurocontrol.int/ehp/?q=Home) supports this process and represents a list of HP activities. It contains standard HP methods, tools, guidelines, and techniques as well as specifically developed tools to support ATM design. These specific tools include, for example, guidelines for addressing HP automation issues (SESAR, 2013a), competence and training assessment (Heintz et al., 2016), and guidance for information presentation (SESAR, 2013b). The following section outlines two of these guidelines.

The Human and the System – Addressing Automation Issues

In the early stages of the SESAR program, it was stated that human operators had to remain at the core of the ATM system, but had to work in an operational environment characterized by a constantly increasing role of automation, considered essential for achieving the ambitious performance targets set by the Single European Sky Initiative (SESAR, 2007a). Therefore, as part of the HP assessment methodology the definition of design principles for HP automation support was considered a very important element. As a result, a specific SESAR project dealing with the "Identification and Integration of Automation Related Good Practices" elaborated on a new conceptual framework to compare different design options and to provide guidance on how to choose among them. The framework consists of a level of automation taxonomy (LOAT) taking the form of a table, with the rows representing different automation levels and the columns representing different psychomotor functions (Save, 2014, 2015; Save & Feuerberg, 2012). The LOAT is grounded on the seminal work by Sheridan and Verplank (1978) – the first to introduce the idea of automation levels – and on the subsequent work by Parasuraman, Sheridan, and Wickens (2000) defining four functions to be supported in a human–machine system: *information/data acquisition, information analysis, decision and action selection,* and *action implementation*. Although the model by Parasuraman and colleagues helped to understand the variable nature of automation support, it was of limited support for the identification of distinctive levels for the classification of SESAR-automated functionalities. The elaboration of the LOAT filled this gap, by combining a theoretical work derived from activity theory and distributed cognition (Hutchins & Klausen, 1996; Nardi, 1996) with the analysis of 26 examples of automated functionalities. Some of them where part of air traffic controller tools, while others were related to the work of pilots.

In its most recent format (Save, 2019), the LOAT table (presented here in a condensed version, Table 1.1) combines the four psychomotor functions mentioned earlier with distinctive automation levels: five levels for information acquisition and information analysis, six for decision and action selection, and eight for action implementation.

In addition, three different clusters group all the levels. In the upper cluster (human), all psychomotor functions are simply under control of the human. In the intermediate cluster (automation support), all functions are supported by automation. Finally, in the third cluster (automatic), all functions are under the direct initiative of automation. The taxonomy helps to classify specific functionalities of the automated system, by analyzing in detail the type of interaction established with the human when performing their specific tasks. For example, the MTCD (medium-term conflict detection) normally has more automated functions incorporated for the air traffic controller. Some of them are activated only on the controller's request, as with the *what-if function* used to anticipate potential conflicts before issuing a clearance. While others automatically trigger an alert as soon as the alerting logic of the tool detects a conflict, with no need for user activation. Both processes are information analysis functions. However, the what-if corresponds to a Level B3 in the taxonomy (lower level of automation), while the functions triggering alerts automatically corresponds to a Level B4 (higher level of automation). There might be cases in which the same automated functionality supports more than one psychomotor function, covering different cells in the taxonomy. For example, the TCAS RA (traffic collision avoidance system – resolution advisory; here, we refer to TCAS II Version 7.1) in its classic implementation plays a double role. It supports decision and action selection at a Level C4, by indicating to the pilot one unique avoiding maneuver to fly in order to avoid collision with another aircraft. Then, it supports action implementation at a Level D2, by providing visual and acoustic feedback to the pilot flying the avoiding maneuver and helping the pilot to understand whether the maneuver is being successful in bringing the aircraft clear of conflict.

The best way to use the LOAT is the four-step methodology indicated in Figure 1.1.

Step 1 requires the identification of a specific proposed automated functionality to analyze. Step 2 scrolls among the columns of the LOAT table to determine the psychomotor function that the automated functionality is supposed to be supporting. Step 3 scrolls among the rows to identify a specific cell, corresponding to a specific level of automation. Finally, Step 4 considers the design principles applicable to the specific level of automation.

These design principles refer to factors such as: the number of information items to be considered by the user, the level of workload associated with the task, the variability and the complexity of the operational environment, the criticality of the task being supported, etc. In the context of industrial projects, it is common to use the term "functions" for what is assigned to automation and "tasks" for what is assigned to the human. This model uses the term "psychomotor function" observing the activities from the perspective of the human operator and assuming that all functions are performed with different levels of cooperation between the human and the automation. But there will of course be other system functions designed to work independently from the supervision or action of a human. The combination of the LOAT table with the design principles allows for the comparison of successful experiences with automation in defined operational contexts with less successful examples, providing more insight into how to prevent HP issues and derive full benefit of the available technical solutions (SESAR, 2013b; for more information on the design principles, the reader is referred to SESAR, 2013a).

From Design to Deployment and Training

Traditionally, attempts to systematically address HF impacts on new developments in aviation, factors such as acceptance, training, or change management have been treated as *impediments* to an innovative technological solution (e.g., HF case Version 1). While much effort was invested in a thorough planning of

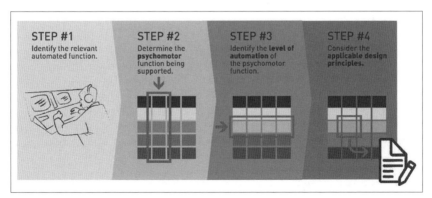

Figure 1.1   The four-step methodology to apply the LOAT. Reprinted with permission from "Un colpevole ci dovra pur essere. I luoghi comuni sugli incidenti e le strategie piu efficaci per evitarli" by L. Save (Ed.), p. 187. © 2019 by Primiceri Editore Italy.

Table 1.1   A condensed version of the level of automation taxonomy (LOAT)

A Information acquisition	B Information analysis	C Decision and action selection	D Action implementation
Human Information acquisition	Human Information analysis	Human Decision-making	Human Action execution
A0 Manual	B0 Manual	C0 Manual	D0 Manual
A1 Supported by artifact	B1 Supported by artifact	C1 Supported by artifact	D1 Supported by artifact
Automation support to information acquisition	Automation support to information analysis	Automation support to decision-making	Automation support to action implementation
A2 With user filtering and highlighting of relevant info	B2 On user request	C2 With user choice and acceptance among proposals	D2 With user activation and control of actions
A3 With user control of filtering and highlighting criteria	B3 On user request with alerting mechanism	C3 With user acceptance of one proposal	D3 With user activation and control of action sequence
A4 With user awareness of filtering and highlighting criteria	B4 With user setting of alerting parameters		D4 With user activation, monitoring and interruption of action sequence
A5 With filtering and highlighting criteria not visible to the user	B5 With alerting parameters not visible to the user		

Table 1.1 continued

A Information acquisition	B Information analysis	C Decision and action selection		D Action implementation	
		Automatic Decision-making		Automatic Action implementation	
		C4	With user informed	D5	With user monitoring, modification or Interruption capabilities
		C5	With user informed on request *Always connected to action implementation D5–D8*	D6	With user monitoring and interruption capabilities
		C6	With user not informed *Always connected to action implementation D5–D8*	D7	With limited user monitoring and interruption capabilities
				D8	With no user monitoring nor interruption capabilities

Note. This condensed version of the LOAT table first appeared in Save (2019). It is reprinted here with permission from "Un colpevole ci dovrà pur essere. I luoghi comuni sugli incidenti e le strategie più efficaci per evitarli," by L. Save (Ed.), p. 187. © 2019 by Primiceri Editore, Italy.

developing, financing, and implementing the technical components (software, hardware), upcoming HF aspects or the need to train the operational staff in applying new systems and procedures were and are dealt with mainly in a reactive mode and treated as impediments to a successful implementation. Training demand is often either underestimated or identified only late in the process, or it is overestimated when comparing new procedures with the existing way of working from a current operator's point of view.

To improve this situation, HP-related work and methods in the SESAR program continued toward widening the focus from classic design issues such as HMI or input devices design to the entire spectrum of HP-related activity, including staffing, competence impacts and associated selection and training, as well as social factors and change management (Heintz & Merz, 2012; SESAR, 2007a). As in the EUROCONTROL HF case, the HPAP systematically covers the area of *transition factors*, treating human-related activities like all other requirements to successfully implement a new system or new procedures. In order to enable a timely consideration of these aspects in project management, the arguments in the area of transition factors encompass all steps of analysis and implementation to ensure that the ATM system in the widest sense will ultimately deliver the envisaged performance targets. As ATM is still expected to remain a human-centered activity (SESAR, 2007a; SESAR, 2017a), the arguments related to transition factors aim to bring the planning of staffing and training at the same level as the usual technical and operational deployment sequences.

Thus, the HP assessment process intends to go beyond being a pure design guidance or contributing to an isolated safety assessment. With regard to the overall performance of the aviation system, it also serves to assure key performance indicators (KPIs) such as capacity (e.g., to trigger timely and sufficient staffing), cost efficiency (e.g., through early and consistent integration of training cost and effort), security, and others. Consequently, the human performance assessment process is now fully embedded in the SESAR Performance Framework (SESAR, 2017b).

Challenges to Ensure and Consolidate the Success of Human Performance Assessments: Managing HF Competence?

The HP assessment has become a compulsory element of Europe's largest aviation R&D program and directly contributes to the overall performance framework related to the European ATM Master Plan. While this can be seen as major progress compared with the beginning of HF integration into system design, its consistent and harmonized application needs further work and support, which is a prerequisite for identifying aggregated performance benefits from the HP domain. Given the level of ambition of the ATM Master Plan as well as the potential impacts of upcoming technological developments (e.g., AI, RPAS), the HPAP is at least ready to ensure that HP is systematically addressed even better for future developments.

Still, despite the overall good integration of the HPAP in the program, the experience of SESAR 1 has demonstrated that many challenges remain that HF specialists need to overcome in order to better integrate HF in technical projects (Biede-Straussberger & Pelchen-Medwed, 2017). Having access to HF competence brought by HF specialists as part of the program is only a starting point. But, as already reflected in the SESAR arguments, the HF topics to be covered are very diverse, whereas the competence of available HF specialists is often specific. They come from various backgrounds, such as operational or engineering training with additional HF training, or specific human sciences studies such as psychology, linguistics, physiology, or others. This raises a new question about the identification and management of the adequate HF competence needed within projects. In the airborne industry, managing HF competence resulted in introducing HF specialists not only as part of the cockpit, cabin, and cargo design and maintainability, but moreover also in in-service event analysis, training efficiency, and manufacturing. Such a type of reflection can be extended to the wider ATM system, in order to find the adequate mapping between the ATM HF topics and the human sciences academic disciplines. Especially in the context of preparing the future management of HF competence, it is a difficult question not only for an aircraft manufacturer, but for the aeronautical community as a whole. First, the introduction of artificial intelligence components such as machine learning, natural language processing, human monitoring systems, image processing, or robotics, combined with the emergence of new operational concepts (more autonomous vehicles or seamless integration of drones in ATM), increasingly raised questions about the need also for a timely introduction of new competences and insights into neurosciences, neuro-ergonomics, etc. Second, the deep transformation of operators' roles and its impact on society also requires specific competencies in anthropology, sociology, digitalization, and big data.

Having recruited some HF competences is a good starting point, but additional actions are needed to integrate these competencies into different expertise teams located near the applications and being part of a multidisciplinary integrated team with system designers, operations, and HMI designers, etc. Further emphasis shall be given to organize HF competence in the processes and governance of the company to structure and legitimate the different HF activities, being accompanied by dissemination of HF knowledge following HF training and awareness plans (Reuzeau, 2019). Whereas SESAR has already largely achieved the latter by ensuring the integration of HF in the program's process handbook followed by projects, the real integration of HF competencies throughout the project lifecycle as well as a smooth and efficient association of local company processes with SESAR requirements remains to be fully established. Even though several guidance documents and tools have been established in the program to harmonize collaboration in design, training, and social impacts, only by ensuring a recognized, empowered, and strongly embedded HF competence linked across organizations and industries will future HP benefit to the full extent.

References

Ahlstrom, V., & Longo, K. (2003). *Human factors design standard (HF-STD-001)*. Federal Aviation Administration.

Biede-Straussberger, S., & Pelchen-Medwed, R. (2017). *Effectiveness of the application of the human performance assessment process in SESAR 1. Sharing lessons learnt.* Proceedings of the 12th USA/Europe Air Traffic Management Research and Development Seminar. http://www.atmseminar.org/12th-seminar/papers

Chalon-Morgan, C., Pelchen-Medwed, R., Dehn, D., Maddalena, C., Pinheiro, J. P., & Josefsson, B. (2012). Development of an argument and evidence based human performance assessment process for SESAR. In A. Droog (Ed.), *Proceedings of the 30th conference of the European Association for Aviation Psychology* (pp. 247–253). European Association for Aviation Psychology.

EUROCONTROL. (1999). *Programme for harmonized air traffic management research in EUROCONTROL, PHARE final report, Doc 99-70-09*. https://www.eurocontrol.int/phare/gallery/content/public/documents/99-70-09pharefinal10.pdf

EUROCONTROL. (2007). *The human factors case: Guidance for human factors integration edition 2.0*. https://www.skybrary.aero/bookshelf/books/4556.pdf

European Aviation Safety Agency. (2007, September). *Certification specifications for large aeroplanes CS-25 Amendment 3*. https://www.easa.europa.eu/sites/default/files/dfu/CS-25_Amdt%203_19.09.07_Consolidated%20version.pdf

Federal Aviation Administration. (2013, May). *25.1302-1 – Installed systems and equipment for use by the flightcrew*. Responsible Office ANM-111, Northwest Mountain Region, Transport Airplane Directorate.

Heintz, A., Lévêque, I., Georg, W., Biede, S., Leoff, T., & De Beaufort, A. (2016). Interdisciplinary training for task and responsibility shifts in future operational ATM procedures and systems. In M. Schwarz & J. Harfmann (Eds.), *Proceedings of the 32nd conference of the European Association for Aviation Psychology* (pp. 158–179). European Association for Aviation Psychology.

Heintz, A., & Merz, W. (2012). Completing the picture – including human performance impacts related data into SESAR cost benefit analysis and regulatory impact assessments. In A. Droog (Ed.), *Proceedings of the 30th conference of the European Association for Aviation Psychology* (pp. 261–268). European Association for Aviation Psychology.

Hutchins, E., & Klausen, T. (1996). Distributed cognition in an airline cockpit. In D. Middleton & Y. Engeström (Eds.), *Communication and cognition at work* (pp. 15–34). Cambridge University Press. https://doi.org/10.1017/CBO9781139174077.002

Ministry of Defence. (2015). *Human factors integration process (HFI process), Version 1.0.* https://assets.publishing.service.gov.uk/government/uploads/system/uploads/attach ment_data/file/483177/20151030-JSP_912_Part_2_DRU_version_Final-U.pdf

Nardi, B. A. (1996). Activity theory and human-computer interaction. In B. A. Nardi (Ed.), *Context and consciousness: Activity theory and human-computer interaction* (pp. 69–103). MIT Press. https://doi.org/10.7551/mitpress/2137.001.0001

Parasuraman, R., Sheridan, T. B., & Wickens, C. D. (2000). A model for types and levels of human interaction with automation. *IEEE Transactions on Systems, Man, and Cybernetics –Part A: Systems and Humans, 30,* 286–297.

Reuzeau, F. (2019). The key drivers to set up a valuable and sustainable HOF approach in a high-risk company as Airbus. In B. Journé, H. Laroche, C. Bieder, & C. Gilbert (Eds.), *Human and organisational factors: Practices and strategies for a changing world* (pp. 31–39). Springer Nature. https://doi.org/10.1007/978-3-030-25639-5_5

Save, L. (2014). *Not all or nothing, not all the same: Classifying automation in practice. EUROCONTROL Hindsight 20.* EUROCONTROL. https://www.eurocontrol.int/pub lication/hindsight-winter-2014

Save, L. (2015, June). *The right automation in the right context. A conceptual and methodological framework for human performance automation support.* Poster presented at the Eurocontrol_ERA Operational Safety Forum 2015, Brussels, Belgium.

Save, L. (2019). *Un colpevole ci dovra pur essere. I luoghi comuni sugli incidenti e le strategie piu efficaci per evitarli* [There must be a culprit. The clichés of accident causation and how to prevent them]. Primiceri Editore.

Save, L., & Feuerberg, B. (2012). Designing human-automation interaction: A new level of automation taxonomy. In D. De Waard, K. Brookhuis, F. Dehais, C. Weikert, S. Röttger, D. Manzey, S. Biede, F. Reuzeau, & P. Terrier (Eds.), *Human factors: A view from an integrative perspective.* Proceedings of the HFES Europe Chapter Conference, Toulouse, France. http://hfes-europe.org

SESAR Consortium. (2007a). *SESAR definition phase. The ATM target concept D3 (DLM-0612-001-02-00a).* http://www.atmmasterplan.eu

SESAR Consortium. (2007b). *SESAR definition phase. WP 1.7 – D3 human resources (DLW-0612-017-00-1.0).* http://www.atmmasterplan.eu

SESAR Consortium. (2009). *SESAR definition phase D5 – The European ATM master plan, Edition 1.* http://www.atmmasterplan.eu

SESAR Joint Undertaking. (2013a). *Guidelines for addressing HP automation issues, WP 16.05.01 – deliverable 04.*

SESAR Joint Undertaking. (2013b). *Updated generic SESAR information presentation guide; 16.05.03, D06, edition 00.01.00.*

SESAR Joint Undertaking. (2016). *SESAR human performance assessment process V1 to V3 – including VLDs; 16.06.05 D27, edition 00.01.00.*

SESAR Joint Undertaking. (2017a). *SESAR 2020 concept of operations Edition 2017. Report D 19.2.1.*

SESAR Joint Undertaking. (2017b). *PJ 19: Performance framework. Report D4.1PJ 19 CI.*

Sheridan, T. B., & Verplank, W. (1978). *Human and computer control of undersea teleoperators*. Man-Machine Systems Laboratory, Department of Mechanical Engineering, MIT. https://doi.org/10.21236/ADA057655

Chapter 2

The Challenge of Bridging the Gap Between Research and Industrialization: What Human Factors Methodology Can Do

Cedric Bach and Sonja Biede-Straussberger

Abstract

In the literature and international standards, a wide variety of human factors (HF) tools and methods exist that can be applied to ensure the integration of HF in design. Often these methods have been developed and promoted within research environments and are being transposed to industrial settings. The industrial context, however, does not always facilitate their application, due to constraints inherent to industrial environments. These constraints are even reinforced when multiple industries and operators are involved, as is the case in the currently ongoing transformation of air transportation and air traffic management. The goal of this chapter is to provide an overview of existing classification schemes to support the selection of the most adequate methods. Currently applied classification criteria have limitations in addressing the complexity inherent in the design of future systems. The so-called human-oriented approach of interactions with complexity is proposed for a systematic organization of HF methods. It ensures that spatial, temporal, and social units are captured so as to more easily support the identification of appropriate or suitable HF methodology.

Keywords: design methods, classification, industrialization tools, constraints, validation, tools

Introduction

In the literature and international standards, a wide variety of human factors (HF) tools and methods exist. They are recommended to be applied to ensure the integration of HF in product design. Often these methods have been developed and promoted within research environments and are then directly transposed to industrial settings. These settings, however, do not always facilitate their application due to constraints inherent to industrial environments. Such constraints are even reinforced when multiple industries and operators are involved, as is the case in the ongoing transformation of air transportation into future air traffic management (ATM). As a consequence, new challenges arise related to the choice of HF methods that can be compliant with industrial environments.

The goal of this chapter is to provide an overview of existing criteria to classify methods and tools addressing product design and validation phases. However, the increase in complexity in the aviation field envisions an evolution of these classification criteria to incorporate this aspect. This chapter proposes a sense-making framework able to characterize the required HF activities leading to a new classification method in accordance with the complexity of future operational concepts.

State of the Art of HF Methods and Tools

The aim of any method is to be shared and used for the design of sociotechnical systems. Today, several standards (e.g., International Organization for Standardization [ISO], 2002), handbooks, and web references (e.g., SESAR HP repository, https://ext.eurocontrol.int/ehp/) propose a set of HF methods dedicated or not to the aviation domain. These methods and knowledge were developed and structured over the years. One of the first handbooks to structure HF knowledge was published in 1949 by Tufts College (Tufts, 1949) for the US Navy. In the same year, Chapanis et al. (1949) published their first textbook on *Human Factors in Engineering Design* in the open literature, followed by a first compilation and structured approach of HF for aeronautics by Fitts and colleagues in 1951 dealing with topics such as the design of air traffic control (ATC) systems; visibility of displays/cockpit/runways; man/machine task allocation; decision-making; and voice communication. The field of HF and ergonomics evolved along with the technological progress, for example, the introduction of glass cockpits in the 1980s (Wiener, 1989), and resulted in the publication of a HF training manual by the International Civil Aviation Organization (ICAO) in 1998. The latter includes in its first part the presentation of HF concepts and a general presentation of HF methods dedicated to different domains such as the flight crew, ATC, as well as aircraft maintenance and inspection. The second part proposes a backbone of training programs for operational personnel.

During the 1990s, with personal computing and the introduction of human–computer interaction, the concept of usability became more popular within the discipline of industrial HF. The Association for Computing Machinery (ACM) created the Special Interest Group in Computer Human Interaction (SIGCHI) in 1982 and research on human–computer interactions grew rapidly. The concept of user-centered design is strongly linked to the concept of human–computer interaction and became a standard in 2000 with the publication of the ISO/TR 18529 on the *Ergonomics of Human-System Interaction – Human-Centered Lifecycle Process Descriptions* (this standard has been updated to ISO/FDIS 9241-200 *Ergonomics of Human-System Interaction – Part 220: Processes for Enabling, Executing, and Assessing Human-Centered Design Within Organizations*). Once this process had been standardized and broadcast, a second standard was provided to support this process with the appropriate methods according to different criteria. This standard is named ISO/TR 16982:2002 *Ergonomics of Human-System Interaction – Usability Methods Supporting Human-Centered Design*. It proposes a way of classifying methods as well as a process of choosing them appropriately according to a set of criteria. The introduction of the usability concept and the emergence of personal computing represented an important turning point in the history of aeronautics because the combination of glass cockpits and human–computer interaction opened new perspectives in the way of designing cockpits.

In the same way, since the 1980s the number of HF methods available has grown significantly. In 2005, Stanton et al. (2005) referenced more than 200 HF methods. Therefore, the question of classifying them in order to facilitate their choice became essential. Table 2.1 lists ways of classifying the different types of methods. They are supported by a set of criteria for choosing a relevant method for a defined expectation (e.g., cost efficiency). Some of them are specific to a certain domain and others are common to several domains.

ISO/TR 16982 proposes a set of 24 types structured into six categories able to identify the most relevant method in a set of 12 method types dedicated to usability management. Stanton et al. (2005) provide a review of HF methods cross application domains. The European SESAR program classifies the methods useful for the improvement of European ATM, which also includes concept deployment phases.

Table 2.2 lists the main criteria used to describe, classify, and choose the methods, ranging from a more generic to a more precise description.

Since each type of characterization is limited by definition, it is in fact the combination of both types of approaches, completed by a perspective on complexity, that facilitates the evolution of social–technical environments. They provide a complete although very simplified approach for facing industrial HF challenges in an evolving society, which is developed further in the rest of the chapters in this volume.

Table 2.1   Comparison of method type or category classification between a handbook, SESAR, and the 16982

Stanton's HF handbook	SESAR HP repository	ISO/TR 16982
Data collection techniques Task analysis techniques Cognitive task analysis techniques Charting techniques Human error identification (HEI) techniques Mental workload assessment techniques Situation awareness measurement techniques Interface analysis techniques Design techniques Performance time prediction/assessment techniques Team performance analysis techniques	Organizational implementation of HP • *Identification of competence requirements* • *Identification of selection and training needs* • *Identification of staffing requirements* • *Identification of relevant social factors* • *Identification of issues in change and transition management* Human performance in the working environment • *Design of working environment* • *Assessment of operator working positions* • *Assessment of technical equipment (input devices, visual displays etc.)* Impact on human performance • *Assessment of workload* • *Identification of potential human error and assessment of human error* • *Assessment of trust in systems solution level* • *Assessment of team work and communication* • *Assessment of situational awareness* • *Acceptance* • *Performance measurement* Technical system supporting human performance • *Identification of task allocation between human and machine* • *Identification of human-machine transition issues*	User observation Measurement of performance Critical incident analysis Questionnaires Interviews Thinking aloud Collaborative design and evaluation Creativity methods Document-based methods Model-based approach Expert evaluation Automated evaluation

Table 2.2   Sets of criteria for qualifying and selecting different methods

	Stanton's HF handbook	SESAR HP repository	ISO/TR 16982
General organization	Procedure and advice	General description	General description of methods types
	Flowchart	Technical description of method or tool	
Selection criteria		Applicability to lifecycle (E-OCVM)	Step in the product life cycle (5)
			User characteristics (3)
			Characteristics of the task to execute (6)
			Product or the system itself (3)
			Project environment constraints (5)
	Application time	Required effort to conduct the analysis	Limited time
		Cost information/ copyright/ agreements	Budget control
			High-quality product
			Precocious diagnosis
			Evolutive requirements
			Level of expertise in HF available in the design or evaluation team (2)
	Approximate training	Level of HF expertise needed	HF expertise available
		Usability of the method	HF expertise not available

Table 2.2   continued

	Stanton's HF handbook	SESAR HP repository	ISO/TR 16982
		Requires additional user qualification	
Application criteria	Advantages	Evaluation advantages	Advantages
	Disadvantages	Evaluation disadvantages	Disadvantages
		Constraints concerning conditions of use	Constraints
Descriptive criteria	Name and acronym	Name of the method	
	Author(s)	References	
	Background and applications	Experiences of use by SESAR partners	
	Domain of application	Application area	
	Example	Reported experiences of use; Abstract	
	Related methods	Type of the method	
		Alternative methods	
	Reliability and validity	Reliability/validity	
	Tools needed	Technical requirement for using the method	
		Measure/response type	
		Results obtained and interpretation	

Note. Numbers in parentheses list the number of detailed criteria available.

Specificities of Industrial Environments in Aviation

Users of industrial aeronautical products are not only directly interacting with a product, but they are also members of an organization, selected and trained, and disposing of a certain level of experience. Thus, HF methods should allow one to: access the information on user needs associated with operational and human characteristics, to validate and verify that products will correspond to user needs in addition to further industry-specific needs, and assess that users are able to deliver the expected performance. In order to characterize development cycles, industry has found a way to describe the maturity of products under development in the form of technology readiness levels (TRLs), which are supported by a set of operational and technical criteria (Héder, 2017). Within SESAR HPAP (Biede & Pelchen-Medwed, 2017), these criteria were further extended to include human performance, and support is provided to use the adequate HF method to manage the risks for a targeted level of maturity. But HF methods have often been elaborated within academic contexts and research projects to gain knowledge on why and how the user is interacting with a product, whereas the application of HF methods during industrial developments is exposed to a number of additional challenges described hereafter.

Complexity of Products and Operational Environments

Aviation products, whether at air or ground level, have developed toward a high level of complexity over the past decades to achieve the highly performing operations of today. At the same time, operators' roles have changed, adding further challenges for the engineering and maintenance of such products. This goes together with a multifaceted industry run by multinational collaborations and supplier–manufacturer relationships that are characterized by extended enterprises and partnerships throughout the field. Furthermore, new technologies for data exchange modify information management and communication while still enhancing product performance.

The global evolution of the product (e.g., autonomous vehicles) and of operational environments (e.g., high increase in traffic due to societal demands) also has an impact on how to deal with HF methods. Methods are applied to the development of new products or to enhance existing products. The challenge that remains is the selection of the appropriate method in order to achieve a proper understanding of the user during operations. Consequently, the evolution of a product in aviation cannot be viewed as simply remaining focused on the product, but also requires taking an extended view of the context of use of the product. For HF methods, this enforces seeing not only the direct user–product interaction, but also new underlying issues that may emerge in a multiuser organization–product environment.

Project and Product Lifecycle

Due to the complexity of the context of use, aeronautical evolution and product development need to be long-lasting, especially when several types of operations or organizations are impacted. The evolution of technology also facilitated more rapid iterations and introduced agile developments to industry. This led to additional dynamics, where projects no longer evolved in as linear a manner as in the past, which also had an impact on the application of HF methods.

Thus, in this mixed project landscape between long- and short-lasting developments, the challenge is to identify how to manage HF within a global framework and be able to select quickly the adequate HF method by trained professionals. This is especially true, since the application of HF methods is often perceived, especially by non-HF specialists, as causing delay or being too time-consuming. In fact the issue is more related to a project management matters between system, operational, and HF studies on the one hand, and an oversimplification of the needs of human users by non-HF specialists on the other hand. This may even lead to projects collapsing into chaos (Snowden & Boone, 2007). Consequently, HF methods are required to be adaptable and easily re-scope-able and to easily add comprehensible value by non-HF specialists.

Also, long-lasting projects are usually associated with a certain amount of turnover. As it takes a long time to develop and integrate HF competence in aeronautics, the management of turnover is critical for performance in projects. This raises a dilemma for the application of HF methods, where long-lasting projects are run in an iterative way and subjected to project decision points, but there is little time to produce HF results to support project decisions. This requires a strategic vision and adequate resources for managing HF at the same time as being tactically efficient.

Finally, teams are collaborating over geographically and organizationally different sites. This imposes additional challenges, as HF methods may need to be applied in just such distributed working environments, with HF specialists being trained on the specificities of the industrial environments and their associated soft skills in order to facilitate the adaptation of HF methods therein.

People

Finally, HF is all about people, albeit the human dimension is difficult to grasp in all its scope and details. HF is applied to optimize products, to make them safe and efficient to use from a human perspective. But ensuring HF integration in products also requires knowledge at a professional level and being familiar with the variety of existing HF methods and how to apply them in the context at hand. Furthermore, it requires a global understanding of the complexity of working with project teams as well as the surrounding aeronautical context, in order to select the appropriate methodology for that project.

However, humans have well-known tendencies to bias information in order to efficiently achieve their goals (Tversky & Kahneman, 1974). For example, the perception of the user task is quite evident for user representatives, but subject to biases by engineers or designers. When system designers access information on how users behave, knowledge based on only a few users may be inadequately generalized toward a user population. A significant added value of HF methods consists in controlling for these biases.

The educational landscape for HF specialists requires a better fit with such industrial environments. At entry-level, HF specialists do have profound knowledge on human characteristics and how to access them thanks to studies in psychology, ergonomics, or similar sciences, but training is scarce to prepare for the requirements of a multi-faceted evolving industry. Finally, diversity in concepts and training programs over geographical regions and national levels do not facilitate a common understanding on HF requirements. Hence, the development of initiatives to jointly profit from past lessons learnt is key for the evolution of the HF applications.

Prospect for HF Methods

Within this context of design for future operations and systems, the challenge for HF is to harness HF methodologies within a project team. Indeed, the complexity of the operations is a dimension and an approach to designing human–system integration efficiently (Boy, 2017), an area that needs a dedicated set of HF methods. Complexity must be clearly distinguished from complicated contexts (Snowden & Boone, 2007). In association with future ATM, complexity has its own indicators such as the increased number of agents in line with the increase in traffic and the use of air/ground data exchanges as well as network technologies. Nevertheless, in order to be successful, a complex system must still be understandable and compatible with human capabilities otherwise this might jeopardize its acceptability. To this end the HF field must harness the system's complexity. In fact, the current criteria for classifying HF methods such as the ISO 16982 are quite limited for globally addressing complexity, as they remain focused on the usability and especially the interaction between the *users*, the *products*, and the *tasks to accomplish*.

To completely address complexity, these criteria may also integrate the interactions between humans and the *organizations* and the *environment* in which the action has taken place, such as the airspace, airports, runways, air traffic control centers, airline operation centers, and all the systems linked to these systems. Several authors have already described the complexity of interactions in aeronautics, having identified the components and the interactions between them as a field for the emergence of complexity. Figure 2.1 illustrates the different components interacting with each other. These components are the *users*, the *artifacts/human machine interface (HMI)*, the *environments/situations*, the *organizations*, and the *tasks to accomplish* as a link between the components (see Barbé & Boy 2006; Perret et al., 2016; Ragosta et al., 2015). The relationships between these components can refer to: (1) the task and activity requirements such as the goals, action level, user's experience level; (2) the information and technological requirements such as the automation and/or computerization level; (3) the human organization requirements such as the responsibility, authority, role, operational procedure, training; and (4) the adaptability requirements such as the level of adjustment and temporal constraints.

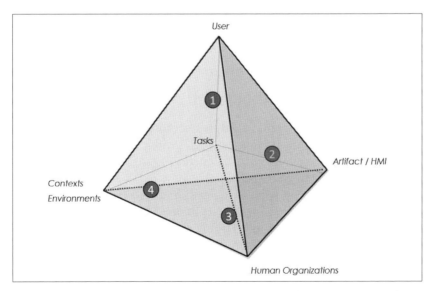

Figure 2.1   Illustration of the interacting components of aeronautical complexity. Adapted from Perret et al., 2016.

The purpose of this section is to present a structured view of a human-oriented approach of interactions with complexity (HOAC). It presents a theory providing a matrix that develops the design and evaluation of interactions dealing with complexity and reflects the organization of methodologies harnessing complexity. A detailed description of this matrix is available for the interested reader in the work of Bach et al. (2017).

Layers to Understanding Human-Oriented Interactions With Complexity

Complex systems have multiple agents that execute actions in collaboration and cooperation with other entities. The organization of these entities needs to be described in detail to understand the wide-ranging impact of agent actions. Actions can be conducted by human or technical agents that belong to the same or to different spatial, temporal, or social units. These units can be characterized along layers ranging from a detailed nano layer to a high-level macro layer. This differentiation is quite common in different domains such as economy, sociology, as well as ecology. However, additional levels were required for complex interactive systems and have been previously described in the field of incident reports (Winckler et al., 2013) and adapted to the context of authority-sharing in ATM by introducing a nano layer (Henry et al., 2015).

In line with the concept introduced by Bronfenbrenner (1979), the micro layer covers a pattern of activities and roles in a specific context and can be understood as linked to an individual unit; the meso layer addresses a setting in which an individual engages for a certain amount of time; and the macro layer entails social and cultural values that exert strong influence. The nano layer covers different subsystems engaged at the micro layer, which could be either different aircraft systems or activated cognitive states. An agent may be connected to different layers at the same time. Depending on the layer at which an agent is acting, its impact is different and as a consequence the HF specialist may describe the interaction with complexity through the characteristics and scale of the macro, meso, micro, or nano layer.

For example, if a HF specialist is designing an authority-sharing philosophy between humans and systems, he or she could consider the interaction with an HMI at the micro level and the definition of roles and responsibilities by authorities at a macro level. Along the same lines, the space and time of actions and design are impacted by the different layers. For example, the micro level space and time may be the cockpit and tactical actions, whereas at a macro level the HF specialist should consider the impact of a new concept directly at traffic scale (and not on a single aircraft) with a long-term perspective.

HOAC, a Framework for Human-Oriented Interactions With Complexity

Finally, in order to draw the big picture of HOAC in aeronautics, the layers could be mixed with the pyramid components of Figure 2.1. This is illustrated in Table 2.3 that shows the interaction between the tasks and the vertex of the pyramid: HMI, environment, human organization, and users. The examples are expected to guide the HF specialist in aeronautics to understand more concretely the link between his/her own (daily) activity with the different complexity dimensions of the HOAC framework and consequently derive the choice of the relevant HF methods in line with the level of their intervention. The cells of the matrix elicit different HF activities addressing the interactions with complexity and by extension the different methods and tools supporting these different activities.

Many of the existing methods may be applied to assess the concept across the layers illustrated in Table 2.3. Eye-tracking or algorithm studies elicit a nano level, some usability criteria a micro level, SA methods can mix different levels around the meso level, and finally the traffic simulator may help to facilitate the transition factors at a macro level.

The approach enables the preparation of a systematic organization of HF methods to more easily support the identification of appropriate or suitable HF methodology for a given project phase. If these different dimensions are not considered in the design of a new concept, this may be viewed as a way of oversimplifying the design process and a way to save time in development in the short term, but not managing risks in the long-term.

Conclusion

The HF field has been rapidly populated by an increasing number of methods since World War 2. Today the main challenge for the HF specialist is to choose or identify the appropriate methods according to the characteristics of a project. This is the purpose of the ISO 16982 standard. Nevertheless, the HF domain today faces a challenge heretofore unseen in aviation history. This challenge requires using and adjusting the relevant level of complexity needed to improve overall efficiency of the socio-technical systems. This new challenge is a step ahead from the "simple" usability and requires addressing dimensions such as trust or adaptive man/machine task alloca-

Table 2.3 Examples of instantiations of the combinations in the HOAC matrix – examples of methods/use cases are in square brackets

	Nano layer	Micro layer	Meso layer	Macro layer
1 Task → User	Concrete user actions/inputs for the task execution [eye tracking: physical sensor studies]	Properties of an agent such as its competences, strengths, and weaknesses [user characteristics; personas]	Users acting directly on planning and execution phases of a mission (a flight leg) [situation awareness; workload assessment]	Definition by authorities of user's responsibilities in a task execution or long-term impact of user on task and vice versa [long-term studies]
2 Task → HMI	Concrete execution of components as system function [simulator logs; log files]	Functional model supporting the immediate task execution at a tactical level [task allocation; level of automation]	HMI supporting the mission execution at a leg level (e.g., FMS, ND, display of ATC sector) [usability studies]	Design of HMI interaction philosophy at a manufacturer level [fleet HMI consistency; standard]
3 Task → Organization	Agent may embody different roles and a set of aggregated connected actions [think aloud; activity analysis]	Transfer of responsibility from one agent to another according to defined procedure [task-sharing]	Co-execution, sharing a common set of operations at a mission level (ATC/pilot co-operation, pilot task-sharing) [team situation awareness]	Definition of rules or law structuring the overall inner and inter organizations [role play workshop; intercultural studies]
4 Task → Environment	Concrete and direct action of the environment such as gust or flock of birds [event-based assessment]	Adaptation of the task to the locally sensed environment (constraints due to detected weather, terrain) [cross-wind operations; VFR/IFR transitions]	Adaptation of the mission to the forecasted environment (weather forecast, escape routes) [downstream contextual data]	Study of the impact of task on the overall environment such as fuel consumption and traffic impact [long-term traffic simulator]

Note. ATC = air traffic control; FMS = flight management system; HMI = human monitoring interface; IFR = instrument flight rules; ND = navigation display; VFR = visual flight rules. Adapted from Bach et al. (2017).

tion. In this way the HF field needs an additional approach to renew and classify the HF methods and special dedicated methods to deal with the complexity. In this perspective we propose a sense-making framework able to support the HF specialist decision in her or his methods and assessment strategy choices.

References

Bach, C., Perret, V., & Calvet, G. (2017). An integrated approach of human oriented interactions with complexity. In D. Harris (Ed.), *Engineering psychology and cognitive ergonomics: Performance, emotion and situation awareness. Lecture Notes in Computer Science: Vol. 10275* (pp. 247–265). Springer. https://doi.org/10.1007/978-3-319-58472-0_20

Barbé, J., & Boy, G. (2006, September). *On board system design to optimise energy management*. Paper presented at the European Annual Conference on Human Decision-Making and Manual Control, Valenciennes, France.

Biede, S., & Pelchen-Medwed, R. (2017, June). Effectiveness of application of the human performance assessment process in SESAR 1. In EUROCONTROL (Ed.), *Proceedings of the 12th USA/Europe Air Traffic Management Research and Development Seminar, Seattle, WA* (pp. 313–312). EUROCONTROL. http://www.atmseminar.org/12th-seminar/papers

Boy, G.A. (2017). Human-centered design of complex systems: An experience-based approach. *Design Science, 3*, E8. https://doi.org/10.1017/dsj.2017.8

Bronfenbrenner, U. (1979). *The ecology of human development: Experiments by nature and design*. Harvard University Press.

Chapanis, A., Garner, W.R., & Morgan, C.T. (1949). *Applied experimental psychology: Human factors in engineering design*. John Wiley & Sons. https://doi.org/10.1037/11152-000

Fitts, P.M., Chapanis, A., Frick, F.C., Garner, W.R., Gebhard, J.W., Grether, W.F., Henneman, R.H., Kappauf, W.E., Newman, E.B., & Williams, A.C., Jr. (1951). *Human engineering for an effective air-navigation and traffic control system*. National Research Council, Division of Anthropology and Psychology, Committee on Aviation Psychology.

Héder, M. (2017). From NASA to EU: The evolution of the TRL scale in Public Sector Innovation. *The Innovation Journal, 22*(2), 1–23.

Henry, J., Bach, C., & Biede, S. (2015, September). A framework for designing authority and responsibility into complex sociotechnical systems. In M. Feary, T. Feuerle, C. Gonzalez Rechea, F.J. Saez, C. Johnson, C. Martinie, P. Palanque, A. Pasquini, P. van Leeuwen, & M. Winckler (Eds.), *Proceedings of the 5th International Conference on Application and Theory of Automation in Command and Control Systems, Toulouse, France* (pp. 1–10). ACM. https://doi.org/10.1145/2899361.2899362

International Civil Aviation Organization. (1998). *Human factors training manual*. International Civil Aviation Organization, ICAO Doc 9683.

International Organization for Standardization. (2002). *ISO/TR 16982 Ergonomics of human-system interaction — Usability methods supporting human-centred design*. ISO. https://www.iso.org/standard/31176.html

Perret, V., Bach, C., Calvet, G., & Chevalier, A. (2016, September). A user-centred approach of complexity: Toward development of a method to support simplex systems design. In G. A. Boy (Ed.), *Proceedings of HCI-Aero, Paris, France* (pp. 1–4). ACM. https://doi.org/10.1145/2950112.2964576

Ragosta, M., Martinie, C., Palanque, P., Navarre, D., & Sujan, M. A. (2015, September). Concept maps for integrating modeling techniques for the analysis and re-design of partly-autonomous interactive systems. In M. Feary, T. Feuerle, C. Gonzalez Rechea, F. J. Saez, C. Johnson, C. Martinie, P. Palanque, A. Pasquini, P. van Leeuwen, & M. Winckler (Eds.), *Proceedings of the 5th International Conference on Application and Theory of Automation in Command and Control Systems, Toulouse, France* (pp. 41–52). https://doi.org/10.1145/2899361.2899366

Snowden, D., & Boone, M. E. (2007). A leader's framework for decision making. *Harvard Business Review, 85*(11), 68–76.

Stanton, N. A., Salmon, P. L. A., Walker, G. H., Baber, C., & Jenkins, D. P. (2005). *Human factors methods: A practical guide for engineering and design.* Ashgate.

Tufts College. (1949). *Handbook of human engineering data for design engineers.* Tech. Report N° SDC 199-1-1, Special Devices Center.

Tversky, A., & Kahneman, D. (1974). Judgment under uncertainty: Heuristics and biases. *Science, 18*(4157), 1124–1131. https://doi.org/10.1126/science.185.4157.1124

Wiener, E. L. (1989). *Human factors of advanced technology ('glass cockpit') transport aircraft.* NASA Contractor Report 177528. National Aeronautics and Space Administration.

Winckler, M., Bach, C., & Bernhaupt, R. (2013). Identifying user experience dimensions for mobile incident reporting in urban contexts. *IEEE Transactions on Professional Communication, 56*(2), 97–119. https://doi.org/10.1109/TPC.2013.2257212

Chapter 3
Essential Tools for Safety Culture Development in Air Traffic Management

Michaela Schwarz and Julia Harfmann

Abstract

Since 2010, European air navigation service providers have been mandated by law to regularly assess, monitor, and improve safety culture in their organizations. Safety culture hereby, "reflects the individual, group and organizational attitudes, norms and behaviors related to the safe and efficient provision of air navigation services" (CANSO, 2009, p. 11). With this mandate the regulator aims to guarantee high safety standards in air traffic management (ATM) despite the large increase in traffic volume, high ATM system complexity, and increasing technical automation. Most European air navigation service providers have implemented the EUROCONTROL Safety Culture Measurement Toolkit incorporating a questionnaire and focus group method. This chapter provides a review of the essential tools to assess and further develop safety culture within the ATM industry beyond questionnaire and focus group techniques. The tools include the safety-relevant behavior observation technique, the safety buffer–efficiency–task load assessment, and the subjective critical situation rating scale as well as the systematic debriefing method. The tools were validated for operational ATM staff during several research projects between 2010 and 2016 in cooperation with the University of Graz (Austria) and the Austrian Air Navigation Service Provider. Four essential tools for assessing operational safety culture are presented including instructions on how to use them in an operational environment. The four tools are: (1) the safety-relevant behavior observation technique, (2) the safety buffer–efficiency–task load triangle, (3) the subjective critical situations scale, and (4) the systematic debriefing. Selected empirical results from previous validation studies highlight the relationship between the four tools and the objective assessment of safety culture as an alternative to subjective methods.

Keywords: behavior observation, safety buffer–efficiency–task load trade-offs, safety culture, subjective critical situations scale, systematic debriefing

Introduction

In air traffic management (ATM), the safety culture concept was first applied to partially explain the Milano Linate collision on take-off in 2001 and the Ueberlingen mid-air collision in 2002 (EUROCONTROL, 2008). Both accident investigations found a complex management organization, lack of safety and risk management, and absence of a healthy safety culture as contributing factors in the accidents (Agenzia Nazionale per la Sicurezze del Volo, 2004; Bundesstelle für Flugunfalluntersuchung, 2004). In 2008, the European Organisation for Safety of Air Navigation (EUROCONTROL, 2008, p. 1) published a white paper on safety culture in ATM defining safety culture as, "the way safety is perceived, valued and prioritized in an organization. It reflects the real commitment to safety at all levels of the organization." In 2009 the Civil Air Navigation Services Organisation (CANSO, 2014) recognized safety culture as:

> The enduring value, priority and commitment placed on safety by every person and every group at every level of the organization. Safety culture reflects the individual, group and organizational attitudes, norms and behaviors related to the safe provision of air navigations services. (pp. 10–11)

In 2010 the European Aviation Safety Agency (EASA) mandated the regular assessment and improvement of safety culture as way to evaluate the effectiveness of the existing safety management system (European Commission, 2011, 2014). EUROCONTROL was tasked to support the air navigation service providers (ANSPs) in implementing a standardized safety culture survey process and improvement activities. The EUROCONTROL Safety Culture Measurement Toolkit (Fruhen et al., 2013; Gordon et al., 2007; Mearns et al., 2013; Shorrock et al., 2011) incorporating standard questionnaire and focus groups techniques was recommended as best practice. The questionnaire consisted of a standardized set of questions measuring various elements of safety culture such as management and colleague commitment to safety, staffing and resources, procedures and training, communication, speaking up, learning, involvement, risk handling, and just culture. Over the years the EUROCONTROL questionnaire set was validated with a sample size of more than 10,000 people involved in operations including air traffic controllers (ATCOs), air traffic safety electronics personnel (ATSEPs), meteorologists (METs), and their line managers:

1. ATCOs are responsible for the safe and efficient flow of air traffic from the time the aircraft turns on the engines for departure (ground/tower controller), en route (area controller) until the aircraft approaches an airport (approach or terminal control), and upon arrival at the gate (ground/tower controller).

2. ATSEPs are licensed engineers and technicians responsible for repairing and maintaining technical equipment (navigation, communication, surveillance) relevant to air traffic control.
3. Aeronautical METs explore the past, present, and future state of the atmosphere and the climate system, based on laws of physics and by means of mathematical methods. They are responsible for issuing regular MET reports, trends, and significant weather report for airports, airlines, and private pilots.

How to Use the EUROCONTROL Process

The safety culture assessment process is performed by an independent provider (e.g., university, expert consultancy) in two steps starting with handing out the questionnaire in Step 1 and discussing critical results in focus groups together with operational staff. Results from both questionnaire and focus groups are incorporated into a final report that forms the basis for the organization's safety culture action plan. The process is typically repeated every 3 years to allow enough time for an organization to implement improvement measures.

The Problem Statement

The questionnaire method is a reliable, relatively easy, and cost-effective way to assess and monitor attitudes and opinions about safety in a larger group of operational individuals. However, the method was criticized for being subjective and unrelated to operational safety performance (e.g., number of safety-critical incidents or safety-relevant occurrences). Questionnaire results were often perceived as *high-level* and associated improvement measures were not *tangible* enough for operational staff. Considering that safety culture is one element of a broader organizational culture, safety experts and researchers were looking for alternative methods to assess safety culture in the operational environment.

Objectives of This Chapter

The goal is to demonstrate that objective safety culture assessment tools make safety culture more tangible for operational staff and their managers. In the fulfilment of this goal, four essentials tools that were developed and validated in the operational environment over a period of 6 years are presented. These tools are based on behavior observation techniques linked to subjective rating scales combined with interview and debriefing techniques. All four tools were validated for use in the operational environment and were rated as the preferred method (compared with questionnaire techniques) to assess safety culture by operational staff and managers. Operational staff enjoyed the personal contact with the experts applying the tools and reported they felt more involved and more heard and understood in their every-day issues. The four tools are therefore recommended as essential tools for organizations to assess, monitor, and improve their safety culture. The following sections introduce the tools including guidance on how to apply the tools in practice.

Safety Culture Assessment Tools

Safety-Relevant Behavior Observations (SOBs)

The SOB is based on the action-oriented task observation system (Kallus et al., 1998) consisting of a set of protocol sheets. The cover sheet includes general information (demographics) followed by a comments and operational event log (time stamp and short description of event). The third sheet is related to routine behaviors (operational tasks) associated with the respective occupational role (ATCO, ATSEP, or MET) to be observed. The last sheet is related to a set of proactive safety behaviors (compare Table 3.1) linked to safety culture partly based on nontechnical skills and behavior marker literature originally developed for flight deck and cabin crew observations (Häusler et al., 2004; Helmreich et al., 1995; Klampfer et al., 2001).

Table 3.1   List of safety-relevant behaviors for air traffic controllers

No.	Component	Behavior
1	Safety information/ communication (Informed/reporting culture)	• Explicitly talks about safety • Actively listens to others/listens in on other radio-telephony calls • Explains facts to others • Asks colleague for help/advice • States/shares intentions about future actions • Reads back/confirms information • Double-checks information • Makes an informed decision • Provides task/shift handover • Adheres to standard phraseology • Positive/friendly attitude • Takes notes of information to be remembered • Participates in/calls ad hoc meeting • Reports safety hazard/incident • Completes daily protocol (shift log)

Table 3.1   continued

No.	Component	Behavior
2	Safety leadership (Management commitment/just culture)	• Intervenes/speaks up if action deviates from standard procedure • Delegates tasks to others • Prioritizes tasks • Challenges others about safety
3	Teamwork	• Reviews causal factors with colleague/sector partner • Double-checks/verifies information (flight data, routes, pilot requests) • Helps colleagues/sector partner in demanding situations • Points something out to colleague/sector partner • Reminds colleague/sector partner about open task • Follows instructions from colleague/sector partner without delay
4	Other safety behavior (Learning culture/ risk perception)	• Remains alert and focused on the task (sits upright focused on main displays) • Writes/clicks as speaks, reads as listens (multitasking) • Takes time to consider/think • Resists/ignores peer/management pressure • Monitors/crosschecks information (flight data, label info, requests) • Has a learning conversation • Considers and shares risk of actions
5	Resilient safety behavior (Goal-directed solutions, flexibility, improvisation, access to resources) Schwarz, Kallus, & Jimenez (2015), Schwarz, Kallus, & Gaisbachgrabner (2016)	• Trades goals (capacity/efficiency/customer service) conflicting with safety • Actively plans ahead/coordinates upfront • Takes conditions of colleague into account • Bends standard operating procedures for safety purposes • Invents work around procedure for safety/efficiency reasons • Actively increases safety buffers (defensive controlling) • Takes on a colleague's responsibility temporarily • Consults written/printed/approved documentation (manuals, procedures) • Looks up electronic information
6	Stress management	• Signals others to stand by (until time to respond) • Requests repetition of information ("say again") • Exhibits stress symptoms (gestures, voice, facial, sweating etc.) • Defers phone calls • Self-talk (recites working steps aloud)

Note. Adapted with permission from Schwarz, 2015.

How to Apply SOBs

The list in Table 3.1 of safety-relevant behaviors for ATCOs should be adapted to the working position that will be observed. It is essential that operational people familiar with the working position are involved in the adaptation process. Behaviors that will not occur or that occur rarely or cannot be objectively observed at all should be removed from the list, as they will not produce meaningful results.

Behavior observations are usually carried out "over the shoulder" sitting or standing behind or next to operational staff or accompanying operational staff on duty (walking along with them). The position of the observer should be chosen wisely to avoid distractions or hindering operational tasks. The observer should have a good view of the working position including all screens, tools, and equipment used by the operational staff. The list of behaviors should be printed on adequate forms leaving enough space to tally the behaviors occurring over a selected time period. The optimal time period depends on the type of operation. ATCOs, for example, usually are limited to a maximum of 120 min in position and change positions during their shift (executive/planning controller positions, different sectors). Depending on the time of the day (peak traffic, weather conditions, day/night shift), the sector complexity (large sectors, national borders, temporary segregated areas), and the traffic mix (civil/military traffic) shorter or longer observations periods make sense. ATSEPs and METs usually do not have a maximum time in position, but time may be related to certain tasks (e.g., maintaining a piece of equipment, calibrating a tool or system, performing a significant weather observation, creating a meteorological product).

The minimum recommended observation time is 15 min, because the observer needs time to gain awareness of the position he/she is observing and the person observed needs time to forget about the fact that he/she is observed and demonstrates normal (routine) behavior. Behavior observations are always objective and related to the working position and not the individuals manning the working position. In cases of position handovers, the observer remains at the working position for the defined observation period. It is important to stick to the planned observation length and not alter the observation times to achieve comparable results.

It is also necessary to ensure a representative number of observations runs throughout a shift. One observation per working position is not enough to objectify behavior, because people have different working styles. The rule of thumb is to observe at least 25% of staff rotating on one and the same working position to achieve a representative sample and be able to calculate statistical trends.

The behavior observation should be performed by competent and trained observers. Observers must be familiar with the tasks they observe (e.g.,

ATCOs for ATCOs) and must be trained on how to perform over-the-shoulder observations to avoid distracting from or interfering with normal (routine) operations. In the case of non-routine operations (e.g., safety-critical events or emergencies), observations should be stopped and only resumed when operations are back to normal routine. Observations are mentally straining for the observer and require a lot of concentration. Observation windows should therefore be limited to a maximum of 60–90 min depending on the type of operation observed to prevent observer fatigue. Observations should always be voluntary and only performed if operational staff agree to being observed and feel comfortable with the observer/situation. Finally, safety-relevant observations should always be followed up with a postobservational interview allowing for questions and feedback related to the observations. SOBs raw data (tally, absolute frequency of behaviors) may be categorized as variables and entered in statistical programs for further quantitative analysis.

Task Load–Efficiency–Safety Buffer Triangle (TEST)

According to Kallus and colleagues (2010):

> TEST was developed as a new computerized scaling tool for quickly visualizing changes in and trade-offs between the three critical factors that determine the work situation of ATM, i.e. taskload, efficiency and safety-buffers. Based on task analysis of ATM and backed up by the stress-strain model, an easy-to-interpret triangle (Kallus, Barbarino, & Van Damme, 1997) was constructed and validated both in simulated and real ATM workplaces. Results from validation studies showed that TEST does not only reflect the most relevant task characteristics, but also provides additional insights in the controller's working styles. The TEST tool can make ATM safety surveys more efficient and help supervisors to decide about optimal times for opening or closing sectors. (p. 240)

The TEST (Kallus et al., 2010) is used to assess the subjective changes in and trade-offs between task load–efficiency–safety buffer and workload, each rated on a 5-point scale from −2 (= *very low*) to +2 (= *very high*). The TEST is available as an electronic (java) version that can be directly integrated into live or simulator air traffic control exercises as well as in a paper–pencil version. TEST may be integrated with other methods (e.g., safety-related reconstruction interview as well as the behavior observations in life and traffic situations). TEST was originally developed in the ATC environment, but it has also been successfully applied to ATSEPs and METs.

In the ATC environment, task load (T) is associated with traffic load, airspace structure, and traffic complexity. Efficiency (E) considers several parameters such as flight levels, speed, and headings (e.g., direct routings). Safety buffers (S) are generally related to the number of traffic conflicts and minimum distance between aircraft. Depending on the situation, the triangle changes shape and color (from green to red).

In the engineering environment (ATSEPs), task load (T) is associated with the number and complexity of maintenance or incident management tasks (from green to red). Efficiency (E) is related to the number of steps taken to find a problem and solve it or complete a maintenance task. Safety buffers (S) for ATSEPs are related to always being three errors away from a technical malfunction or problem, having multiple redundant systems available, in case something goes wrong.

In the MET environment, task load (T) is associated with the number of weather products over a certain period, the complexity and predictability of the weather situation (significant weather, sudden/unexpected weather changes), or the number of pilots or clients asking for a weather briefing. Efficiency (E) is related to the number of parameters considered to produce a weather product and the accuracy of the forecast. Safety buffers (S) in the MET environment are usually related to the lead time of significant weather forecasts (turbulence, icing, crosswinds, thunderstorms) and the number of parameters considered.

How to Apply TEST

TEST is generally used in relation to the subjective critical situation (SCS) scale (see next section). The electronic TEST version (Java based) may be installed and displayed on support systems or portable electronic devices (smartphones, tablet PCs). Operational staff are prompted to rate their task load, efficiency, and safety buffer at a specific point in time. The rating is done by physically clicking on the triangle and changing the shape of the triangle (clicking on the edges of the triangle and moving the triangle on the screen). In the paper–pencil version, the participant simply marks the appropriate point on a scale. The electronic version uses a *traffic light system* (green, amber, red) to visualize positive (green) and negative (amber, red) trade-offs (see Figure 3.1). In the paper–pencil versions the color must be applied manually based on the predefined cut off scores.

TEST is an easy way to visualize trade-offs and goal conflicts and correlates with safety culture survey results and safety performance. It can be used during training as well as on the job.

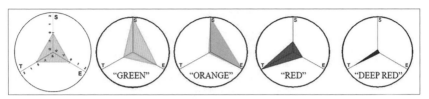

Figure 3.1 Examples of different task load–efficiency–safety buffer trade-offs (TEST electronic version). Reprinted with permission from Schwarz, 2015.

Subjective Critical Situations (SCS) Rating Scale

This scaling procedure was developed based on the category-splitting procedure, which was originally proposed in 1985 by Heller (1991) for the scaling of noise. Participants are asked to rate operational situations on a 50-point scale divided into five subcategories (10 points per category). In general, situations that have an immediate effect on the safe provision of an ATM service (e.g., technical equipment failure, significant weather conditions, and/or unexpected events) are considered as safety relevant. Table 3.2 shows the SCS rating and the associated safety-critical situations in the ATM environment based on real-life examples provided by air traffic controllers.

How to Apply SCS

SCS is typically used in combination with safety-related reconstruction interviews or debriefing of safety-relevant situations. It was initially developed as a paper-pencil version but may also be transferred to electronic tools. On the basis of their rating on the 50-point scale, participants can be subdivided into those who had only routine situations, those who had unusual situations, and those who had critical situations (Kallus et al., 2008) for further evaluation. Based on the scores, associated debriefing sessions may be organized. It is recommended to organize debriefing sessions with persons who experienced subjective safety-critical situations rated higher than 30 (on a 50-point scale).

Table 3.2   Absolute frequency of SCS ratings and associated situations

SCS category	SCS rating	Described situation (example tower/approach control)
Near critical	41–50	• Lost communication/lost radar target • Conflicting taxi clearance • Pilot violations of safety-relevant clearances
Strong deviation	31–40	• Smoke in cabin on ground → fire brigade • Unpredictable weather, very reduced aircraft rate
Deviation	21–30	• Aircraft turned back due to technical problem • Low capacity/delays/slotting due to weather • All aircraft in holding due to weather
Small deviation	11–20	• Low-visibility procedures in the morning • Private jet 45 min in holding due to fog • First shift after 20 days' leave • Many aircraft in holding due to snow • Several missed approaches due to low visibility • Training flight on runway not in use • No visual reduction due to weather
Routine	0–10	• Low traffic • No significant weather conditions • Standard missed approaches • Reduced staffing/scheduled overtime • No VFR/no military traffic, just airliners • All runways in use

Note. SCS = subjective critical situation; VFR = visual flight rules. Reprinted with permission from Schwarz, 2015.

Systematic Team Debriefing

Debriefings are used in numerous high-risk environments, such as the military, the oil and gas industry, aviation, and healthcare. EUROCONTROL suggests using team debriefing for the purpose of learning from incidents not only at a unit level but also at an organizational level (2016):

> The primary aims of the incident debriefing are to understand what happened, to learn from this, and to implement the lessons learned at team level with the objective of preventing the incident from happening again. It is important that the debriefing be conducted as an open and "blame-free" discussion, consistent with a Just Culture philosophy. Each team member should be allowed and encouraged to express their point of view. Feedback to individuals should be constructive – "what would you do differently next time" – not critical or directive ("don't make that mistake again").

Table 3.3 summarizes techniques from different high-risk environments.

Table 3.3   Overview of systematic debriefing techniques

Technique	Authors	Origin	Goal
After action review (AAR)	Department of the Army (1993)	Military operations	Assesses the effectiveness of battle-focused training situations in the military. Formal: focus on good planning, coordination, and preparation (before an event) Informal: focus on intended training objectives, soldier, leader, and unit performance during or immediately after an event.
Guide Team Self-Correction	Smith-Jentsch et al. (2008)	Military operations	Focused on learning from specific situations and use this knowledge in a more general and broader field: "Did we make the right decisions, using processes that across different circumstances increase our odds of success?"
Critical Incident Stress Debriefing (CISD)	Mitchell (1983), O'Flaherty (2006)	Firefighters and para-medics	Coping with traumatic work experiences
Critical Incident Stress Management (CISM) 1:1 Debriefings	Mitchell (1983)	Aviation	Transfer to aviation: CISM aiming at reducing critical incident stress reactions and making operational staff fit for work again, structured intervention/talk about their experiences and get information about their normal reactions to abnormal situations
Debriefing with good judgment	Rudolph et al. (2007)	Healthcare	Avoid trainees in healthcare feeling criticized and offended in debriefings when trainers give any kind of negative feedback
Objective structured assessment of debriefing (OSAD)	Arora et al. (2012), Fanning & Gaba (2007, p. 116)	Healthcare	Facilitator-led participant discussion of events, reflection, and assimilation of activities into their cognitions to produce long-lasting learning
SHARP	Ahmed et al. (2013, p. 959)	Healthcare	• Set learning objectives • How did it go? • Address concerns • Review learning points • Plan ahead

Table 3.3   continued

Technique	Authors	Origin	Goal
Meta-analysis	Tannenbaum & Cerasoli (2013, p. 231) Eddy et al. (2013, p. 977)	Various organizational contexts	Debriefings included had to cover the following aspects to be considered: active self-learning, development intent, specific events, and multiple information sources.

How to Use Systematic Debriefings

A structured team debriefing technique leads operational staff through a predefined set of questions when analyzing their individual or team performance, or certain incidents to learn from for the future. The goal is to prevent incidents from happening again so as to improve ATM safety. Successful debriefings enable a strong learning culture. In ATM, operational staff usually work in dyads (e.g., executive controller and planning controller, meteorology observer and forecaster/nowcaster, engineer and service control supervisor). Their performance usually depends on teamwork, which in turn relates to team quality. A high team quality is an important contributor to a stable safety culture. Consequently, Harfmann (2016) aimed to relate structured debriefing to team quality (see Figure 3.2).

An interview regarding debriefing habits in ATM was designed following the objective structured assessment of debriefing (OSAD) categories (Arora et al., 2012) and consisted of 12 open-ended questions. The first question is an ice-breaker question. It asks for the personal view of the participant on who they consider their direct team. It is the only question that is not directly related to systematic debriefing but asks for the team size. Six questions are related to the *organization of the debriefing* in daily operations. One question is about the *themes* that are covered during debriefing sessions, two questions examine the *value, goals, and impact of the debriefings*. To end the interview, the participants are asked if they would like to add any topic that seems important to them regarding their debriefing habits.

In general, operational debriefings are recommended as standard after every simulator training session to review the trainee's performance and encourage learning from mistakes. In addition, operational debriefings may be applied following safety-relevant incidents in live operations upon request by either the shift supervisor, the staff member concerned, or a team member. Again, the main objective is to discuss the decisions and actions taken by the crew leading up to the incident and to learn from each other and improve overall safety performance. Another area of application would be following continuous competency assessment checks upon request of the examiner or person under examination, to discuss outstanding results as well as areas for performance improvement.

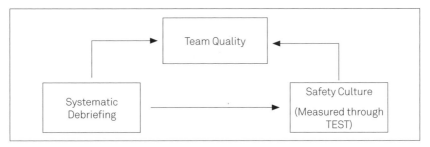

Figure 3.2   Hypothesized relationship between systematic debriefing, team quality, and safety culture. Reprinted with permission from Harfmann, 2016.

Conclusion and Final Remarks

Four essential tools and how to apply them in practice were introduced as alternative to the safety culture questionnaire and focus group techniques. The safety-relevant behavior observation technique (SOBs), the task load–efficiency–safety buffer triangle (TEST), the subjective critical situations (SCS) rating scale, and the systematic debriefing were found to be objective and reliable predictors of the organizational safety culture and safety performance.

Previous studies (Schwarz, 2015) demonstrated that safety-relevant behavior correlated significantly positive with the TEST dimensions safety buffer as well as task- and workload. There was no linear relationship with efficiency. SCS ratings showed moderate correlations with TEST task- and workload. The number of safety-relevant behaviors observed in shift and associated SCS ratings are a stable indicator of an organization's safety culture and broader safety performance.

Harfmann (2016) further suggested that systematic debriefings have a positive effect on safety culture via good teamwork. Management Commitment to Safety was found to be influenced by team debriefings. The debriefing scales Content of Debriefing and Impact of Debriefing correlated positively with Quality of Leadership and Organization of Teamwork. Both team quality scales are influenced by management and safety leadership. That is why it might be beneficial for management to establish a formal debriefing system to increase the staff's perception of management commitment to safety. If the leader tries to cover various topics during the debriefing sessions and focuses on a high impact of the debriefing, it could be supportive to management commitment and proactive behavior by staff. Communication and Learning is also affected by systematic debriefing via high team quality. If systematic debriefing is used as an effective communication tool and the benefits of learning from safety-relevant situations are seen as substantial during the debriefing sessions, this improves the perception of safety culture. There could also be a very practical benefit for the organization since Impact of Debriefing correlates positively with Capacity to Act (in teams). If management installs a well-functioning debriefing system including a high impact it could support the staff's perceptions of their own responsibilities when it comes to safety. Therefore, they may be more likely to share experiences with their colleagues and learn from each other. As Smith-Jentsch et al. (2008) stated, the better teammates know each other and their specific working habits, the more they are willing to accept backup from each other. This means that safety nets could be strengthened through good communication tools such as systematic debriefing.

Overall, participants appreciated the objective tools more than the subjective questionnaire and focus group techniques, because they felt more involved in the safety culture assessment process from the beginning. The list of safety-relevant behaviors was more tangible for them than questionnaire statements regarding safety culture elements (e.g., management commitment to safety, safety reporting and investigation, just culture, training, and procedures etc.) (Schwarz & Kallus, 2015). The objective criteria helped them to recognize safety-relevant behavior in themselves and their colleagues and they were able to relate the somewhat abstract concept of safety culture to their everyday work. No doubt the aforementioned tools presented in this paper require a substantial amount of time and operational resources, as well as trained staff to administer the tools and perform the analysis. In practice, however, each safety culture assessment using the four tools can be considered as a safety culture intervention increasing safety culture awareness and improving an organization's safety performance already during the assessment process.

References

Ahmed, M., Arora, S., Russ, S., Ara, D., Vincent, C., & Sevdalis, N. (2013). Operation debrief: A SHARP improvement in performance feedback in the operating room. *Annals of Surgery, 258*(6), 958–963. https://doi.org/10.1097/SLA.0b013e31828c88fc

Agenzia Nazionale per la Sicurezze del Volo. (2004). *Final report of the Milano Linate Airport disaster*. http://www.ansv.it/cgi-bin/eng/FINAL%20REPORT%20A-1-04.pdf

Arora, S., Ahmed, M., Paige, J., Nestel, D., Runnacles, J., Hull, L., Darzi, A., & Sevdalis, N. (2012). Objective structured assessment of debriefing. *Annals of Surgery, 256*(6), 982–988. https://doi.org/10.1097/SLA.0b013e3182610c91

Bundesstelle für Flugunfalluntersuchung. (2004). *Untersuchungsbericht Überlingen/Boden-see*. [Investigation report Überlingen/Lake Constance]. http://www.bfu-eb.de/EN/Publications/Investigation%20Report/2002/Report_02_AX001-1-2_Ueberlingen_Report.pdf?__blob=publicationFile

CANSO. (2014). *CANSO standard of excellence in safety management systems*. https://www.canso.org/sites/default/files/CANSO%20Standard%20of%20Excellence%20in%20SMS_1.pdf

CANSO. (2009). *The CANSO standard of excellence in safety management systems*. http://www.canso.org/cms/streambin.aspx?requestid=E71C36FB-8804-4FD1-B412-3296E2510EA8

Department of the Army. (1993). *A leader's guide to after-action reviews. Training Circular 25-20*. CreateSpace Independent Publishing Platform.

Eddy, E. R., Tannenbaum, S. I., & Mathieu, J. E. (2013). Helping teams to help themselves. Comparing two team-lead debriefing methods. *Personnel Psychology, 66*(4), 975–1008. https://psycnet.apa.org/doi/10.1111/peps.12041

European Commission. (2011). *Commission implementing regulation (EU) No. 1216/2011 of 24 November 2011 amending Commission Regulation (EU) No. 691/2010 laying down a performance scheme for air navigation services and network functions*. European Commission. http://eur-lex.europa.eu/LexUriServ/LexUriServ.do?uri=OJ:L:2011:310:0003:0005:EN:PDF

European Commission. (2014). *Commission implementing rule 448/2014 of 2 May amending implementing regulation (EU No. 1035/2011)*. European Commission. http://eur-lex.europa.eu/legal-content/EN/TXT/?qid=1418768437844&uri=CELEX:32014R0448

EUROCONTROL. (2008). *Safety culture in air traffic management. A white paper. EURO-CONTROL/FAA as part of the AP15 on Safety Research*. Skybrary. http://www.skybrary.aero/bookshelf/books/564.pdf

EUROCONTROL. (2016). *Incident debriefing*. Skybrary. http://www.skybrary.aero/index.php/Improving_Safety_Culture_in_Air_Traffic_Control#Incident_Debriefings

Fanning, R. M., & Gaba, D. M. (2007). The role of debriefing in simulation-based learning. *Simulation in Healthcare, 2*(2), 115–125. https://doi.org/10.1097/SIH.0b013e3180315539

Fruhen, L. S., Mearns, K. J., Flin, R. H., & Kirwan, B. (2013). From the surface to the underlying meaning – an analysis of senior managers' safety culture perceptions. *Safety Science, 57*, 326–334. https://doi.org/10.1016/j.ssci.2013.03.006

Gordon, R., Kirwan, B., Mearns, K., Kennedy, R., & Jensen, C. L. (2007). A safety culture questionnaire for European air traffic management. In T. Aven & J. E. Vinnem (Eds.), *Risk, reliability, and societal safety. Proceedings of the European Safety and Reliability Conference 2007* (Vol. 2, pp. 1647–1654). Taylor & Francis.

Harfmann, J. (2016). *The relationship between systematic debriefing and team quality in the context of safety culture in air traffic management* (Unpublished master's thesis). University of Graz, Austria.

Häusler, R., Klampfer, B., Amacher, A. & Naef, W. (2004). Behavioral markers in analyzing team performance of cockpit crews. In R. Dietrich, & T. M. Childress (Eds.), *Group interaction in high-risk environments* (pp. 25–38). Routledge.

Heller, O. (1991). Oriented category scaling of loudness and speech audiometric evaluation. In A. Schick, M. Meism & C. Reckhardt (Eds.), *Contributions to psychological acoustics* (pp. 135–159). BIS.

Helmreich, R. L., Butler, R. E., Taggart, W. R., & Wilhelm, J. A. (1995). *Behavioral markers in accidents and incidents: Reference list. NASA/UT/FAA Technical Report 95-1.* The University of Texas.

Kallus, K. W. (2010). *Erstellung von Fragebogen* [Questionnaire Development]. Facultas.

Kallus, K. W., Barbarino, M., & Van Damme, D. (1997). *Model of the cognitive aspects of air traffic control (HUM.ET1.ST01.1000-REP-02). Released issue. Edition 1.0.* EUROCONTROL.

Kallus, K. W., Barbarino, M., & Van Damme, D. (1998). *Integrated task and job analysis of air traffic controllers. Phase 1: Development of methods.* EUROCONTROL, Ref. No. HUM. ET1.1000-Rep-03.

Kallus, K. W., Hoffmann, P., & Winkler, H. (2008, October). The concept of subjective critical situations (SCS). In A. Droog & T. D'Oliveira (Eds.), *Proceedings of the 28th conference of the European Association for Aviation Psychology* (pp. 151–153). EAAP.

Kallus, K. W., Hoffmann, P., Winkler, H., & Vormayr, E. M. (2010). The taskload-efficiency-safety-buffer triangle – development and validation with air traffic management. *Ergonomics: Special Issue on Human Factors in Aviation, 53*(2), 240–246. https://doi.org/10.1080/00140130903199897

Klampfer, B., Flin, R., Helmreich, R. L. Häusler, R., Sexton, B., Fletcher, G., Field, P., Staender, S., Lauche, K., Dieckmann, P., & Amacher, A. (2001, July). *Enhancing performance in high risk environments: Recommendations for the use of behavioural markers.* Workshop at Swissair Training Centre, Zurich, Switzerland.

Mearns, K., Kirwan, B., Reader, T., Jackson, J., Kennedy, R., & Gordon, R. (2013). Development of a methodology for understanding and enhancing safety culture in air traffic management. *Safety Science, 53,* 123–133. https://doi.org/10.1016/j.ssci.2012.09.001

Mitchell, J. T. (1983). When disaster strikes ...the critical incident stress debriefing process. *Journal of Emergency Medical Services, 8*(1), 36–39.

O'Flaherty, J. (2006). Critical incident stress management in airlines. In J. Leonhardt & J. Vogt (Eds.), *Critical incident stress management in aviation* (Chapter 8). Routledge.

Rudolph, J. W., Simon, R., Rivard, P., Dufresne, R. L., & Raemer, D. B. (2007). Debriefing with good judgment: Combining rigorous feedback with genuine inquiry. *Anesthesiology Clinics, 25*(2), 361–376. https://doi.org/10.1016/j.anclin.2007.03.007

Schwarz, M. (2015). *Empirical analysis of safety culture and safety-relevant behaviour and their relationship with organisational resilience and psychological stress in air traffic management.* Unpublished doctoral dissertation, University of Graz.

Schwarz, M., & Kallus, K. W. (2015). Safety culture and safety-relevant behaviour in air traffic management. Validation of the CANSO safety culture maturity concept. *Aviation Psychology and Applied Human Factors, 5*(1) 3–17. https://doi.org/10.1027/2192-0923/a000068

Schwarz, M., Kallus, K. W., & Jiménez, P. (2015). Organisationale Resilienz und Sicherheitsverhalten in der Flugsicherung: Empirische Untersuchung von individuellen und tätigkeitsspezifischen Zusammenhängen [Organisational resilience and safety-relevant behaviour in air traffic management: Empirical analysis of individual and job specific correlations]. In U. Bargstedt, G. Horn, & A. Van Vegten (Eds.), *Resilienz in Organisationen* (pp. 47–62). Verlag für Polizeiwissenschaft.

Schwarz, M., Kallus, K. W., & Gaisbachgrabner, K. (2016). Safety culture, resilient behaviour, and stress in air traffic management. *Aviation Psychology and Applied Human Factors, 6*(1), 12–23. https://doi.org/10.1027/2192-0923/a000091

Shorrock, S. T., Mearns, K. J., Laing, C., & Kirwan, B. (2011). Developing a safety culture questionnaire for European air traffic management: Learning from experience. In M. Anderson (Ed.), *Contemporary ergonomics and human factors 2011. Proceedings of the International conference on Contemporary Ergonomics and Human Factors 2011, Stoke Rochford, Lincolnshire* (pp. 56–63). CRC, Taylor & Francis.

Smith-Jentsch, K. A., Cannon-Bowers, J. A., Tannenbaum, S. I., & Salas, E. (2008). Guided team self-correction impacts on team mental models, processes, and effectiveness. *Small Group Research, 39*(3), 303–327. https://doi.org/10.1177/1046496408317794

Tannenbaum, S. I., & Cerasoli, C. P. (2013). Do team and individual debriefs enhance performance? A meta-analysis. *Human Factors, 55*(1), 231–245. https://doi.org/10.1177/0018720812448394

Chapter 4
Anticipation-Based Methods for Pilot Training and Aviation Systems Engineering

Ioana V. Koglbauer and Reinhard Braunstingl

Abstract

Anticipatory behavioral control is essential for effective human performance in aviation settings such as the prediction and avoidance of collisions, and the management of normal or critical aircraft states. Anticipatory processes allow for proactive action instead of reaction. Anticipation involves a multitude of cognitive processes including learning, cognition, motor control, as well as motivational and emotional processes. In the field of air traffic control, Kallus et al. (1997) modelled anticipative processes involved in critical cognitive work aspects. The anticipation–action–comparison unit emerged that integrates the concepts of situational awareness (Endsley, 1988) and anticipatory behavioral control (Hoffmann, 1993, 2003). This chapter shows how the anticipatory paradigm can be applied to develop pilot training programs. In addition, this chapter describes how engineered systems can support the anticipatory behavior of pilots and air traffic controllers. The final section addresses Butz's (2016) computational theory of cognition and applications to the development of artificial intelligence.

Keywords: anticipatory processes, anticipation-action unit, pilot training, systems engineering, predictive automation, artificial intelligence

Introduction

Pilots and air traffic controllers work in a complex and dynamic environment where safe performance depends on anticipation and timely communication or performance of actions. For example, they cannot simply sit and wait to witness a collision between two aircraft, they must anticipate it and act to prevent it. Anticipation or projection of future changes relevant to operational goals of an individual is considered the highest level of situational awareness (SA; Endsley, 1988). SA has as a prerequisite the perception and understanding of key situational elements and their goal relevance (Endsley, 1988). Fast information processing and SA are enabled by mental models that are activated by sensory cues (Endsley, 2000).

Kallus et al. (1997) interviewed over 100 air traffic controllers to explore their cognitive strategies in developing and maintaining a mental picture of the traffic situation. Interview data were processed using qualitative analyses. The results show that air traffic controllers develop a mental picture of a traffic situation based on expectations (e.g., knowledge, mental models) and real cues. Based on these data, Kallus and colleagues (1997) developed an anticipation-action-comparison model that can predict the maintenance or loss of traffic overview of the controllers in both normal and critical situations (Figure 4.1). The maintenance of the traffic picture requires accurate anticipations of both the system behavior and the effect of control commands. The controllers are continuously checking the match between anticipated and real changes. Every match would reinforce their mental model, but a perceived mismatch would weaken its predictive value and, thus, the use of that particular mental model in a given situation. In a similar manner, the operators predict the effects of their actions based on the perceived situational elements (mental picture) and stored internal models of action. Actual and anticipated action effects are then compared. Every match between anticipated and real effects reinforces their internal model of action, whereas any perceived mismatch weakens the use of that particular model of action in a similar situation (Kallus et al., 1997). The anticipation-action-comparison unit includes elements of both situational awareness (Endsley, 1988, 2000) and anticipatory behavioral control (Hoffmann, 1993, 2003).

The core element of anticipatory behavioral control (ABC) is the internal model of action (Hoffmann, 1993, 2003). Anticipated goal-relevant effects trigger actions (Hoffmann, 2003). In the ABC framework, internal models of action are developed through anticipatory learning mechanisms. It should be noted that anticipatory behavioral control can be initiated by subliminal cues that activate internal stimulus–response associations (Kunde et al., 2003). That is, intentional responses can be linked to stimuli that have never been consciously identified (Kunde et al., 2003). Kallus and Tropper (2007) showed that anticipatory processing in pilots during flight involves both conscious and unconscious mechanisms.

The mismatch between anticipated and actual action effects has been studied by Kallus and Tropper (2007) in pilots performing a "black hole" approach. The group of pilots who crashed had a significantly higher heart rate than the pilots who successfully landed. According to Kallus and Tropper (2007), the pilots who crashed continued the approach instead of go-

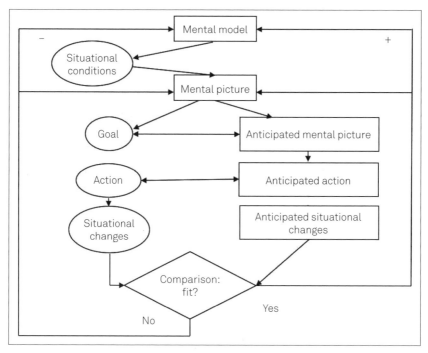

Figure 4.1   The anticipation–action–comparison unit. Reprinted with permission from "Model of the Cognitive Aspects of Air Traffic Control" by K. W. Kallus, M. Barbarino, & V. van Damme (Report No. HUM.ET1.ST01.1000-REP-02), Figure 5. © 1997 EUROCONTROL.

ing-around despite mismatches and an aroused physiological state. This was explained by the nature of anticipative processes that pilots need not be aware of or understand.

Talker and Kallus (2015) also investigated the role of distraction on anticipatory mismatches in pilots with different levels of experience. They studied the effect of inducing the Coriolis illusion (a wrongly perceived pitch-up or pitch-down motion) in a simulator cabin in constant clockwise horizontal rotation. A reaction test was used as a distractor. The participants were asked to push a button when hearing a particular sound sequence. This study showed that the distraction of attention and the connected movement of the head may result in a mismatch between expected and actual sensations of motion. Thus, if experienced pilots fail to anticipate the effect of moving their head while in constant horizontal motion, they are prone to the Coriolis effects (e.g., the illusion of pitching up). Experienced pilots that kept focusing their attention mainly on the ongoing motion had fewer mismatches. Talker and Kallus (2015) concluded that distracting top-down attention from flight affects anticipatory processes negatively, thus, enabling illusions and misperceptions such as the Coriolis effect. As in the study of Kallus and Tropper (2007), mismatches have been found to be accompanied by a specific pattern of physiological activation.

Applications of the Anticipatory Paradigm to Pilot Training

The effect of pilot training on anticipatory processes has been studied extensively (Kallus, 2012; Kallus & Tropper, 2007; Koglbauer et al., 2011; Talker & Kallus, 2015). Applications of the anticipatory processing paradigm to pilot training aim to support trainees in developing mental models and internal models of action that include action–effect relationships. Feedback fosters the comparison mechanism, and the adjustment of mental models and internal models of action.

Collision Avoidance Training

Koglbauer (2015a) developed a method for training student pilots to anticipate the time-to-collision, the relative distance and to select a proper avoidance action during simulated flight including collision and non-collision scenarios. As soon as the trainee decided the encountered traffic was on collision course, the simulation was frozen. The trainee then verbalized an estimation of the time-to-collision and relative distance between their aircraft and the conflicting traffic, as well as the correct avoidance action in accordance with the rules of the air for visual flight rules (VFR) flight. The trainee received immediate feedback about the correct parameters. Estimation accuracy was assessed as the ratio of subjective–to–objective time-to-collision (Koglbauer, 2015b). Thus, a ratio of 1 indicates a match between the subjective estimation and objective measurement. The trainees significantly improved their estimation accuracy: After training the average ratios of subjective–to–objective time-to-collision decreased from 1.97 ($SD=0.28$) to 0.84 ($SD=0.06$). In addition, the average ratios of subjective–to–objective distance improved from 2.16 ($SD=0.31$) to 1.52 ($SD=0.14$). Furthermore, the ability of trainees to select correct avoidance actions improved after training. Koglbauer's (2015a) results show how the anticipative paradigm can be applied to teach anticipatory cognitive skills for collision detection and avoidance. Specific feedback enabled the comparison between anticipated and real collision parameters and an improvement of trainees' predictions and action selection.

Airport Area Approach Training

Another anticipative training method studied combined elements of both traffic and airport procedures (Koglbauer & Braunstingl, 2018). To develop and maintain a mental picture of the traffic situation in the airport area, trainees must develop a mental model of the airport procedures and integrate the actually perceived cues (e.g., verbal ATC communications with themselves and other aircraft, traffic display and communications of other aircraft with ATC). They also need to rotate the mental picture and anticipate their own future position and the future relative positions of other traffic. In the study, the instructor checked participants' comprehension of the ATC clearances by asking the participant to repeat the clearance and, when applicable, to draw the cleared route on a moving map application. Training materials included a naturalistic flight simulation in a network of fixed-based flight simulators with wide-angle multi-channel visual systems. Main features were simulated traffic and radio communication. The trainees could see their own position, a moving airport chart with the traffic pattern, and other aircraft on a tablet PC application (Figure 4.2). This was designed to help the trainees in building a mental picture of the airport and traffic situation. The moving feature of the map assisted the trainees to rotate their mental pictures appropriately and predict the effects of their actions. The trainees were asked to read-back and draw the clearances received from the air traffic controller such as taxi, departure, and approach routes and received immediate feedback from the instructor. For the instructor it was im-

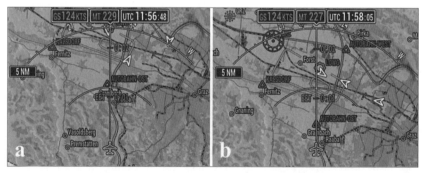

Figure 4.2   The tablet application displays the traffic situation at the airport. The traffic situation in approach changes from a to b. The one's own position is illustrated by an aircraft icon at the bottom of the map display. The position of other aircraft is illustrated by yellow arrows. Reprinted with permission from *Transportation Research Part F: Psychology and Behavior*, Vol. 58, I. Koglbauer & R. Braunstingl, "Ab Initio Pilot Training for Traffic Separation and Visual Airport Procedures in a Naturalistic Flight Simulation Environment," pp. 1–10. © 2018 Elsevier.

portant to see the drawings, because sometimes trainees read-back correctly, but did not understand correctly what they had to do. Clearances included taxiing behind other aircraft, a specific departure clearance to avoid other aircraft in holding, or joining the downwind to land as Number 2. Effects of this anticipation-based training were assessed in a pretest-training-posttest design with 53 ab initio learner pilots assigned to an experimental and a control group. As an outcome of the specific training learners' situational awareness and performance significantly improved in the experimental group, while work strain related to building a mental picture of the traffic situation, airspace monitoring, and coordination with other aircraft had been significantly reduced (Koglbauer & Braunstingl, 2018). The trainees reported that training materials were useful. The anticipation-based training with feedback elements facilitated better understanding, decisions and performance (Koglbauer & Braunstingl, 2018).

Unusual Attitude Recovery Training

A pilot's ability to anticipate can be seen as a top-down process based on a mental model-of-flight situations developed through learning and used to anticipate changes in specific flight situations and the effect of the pilot's specific control actions (Kallus, 2009). Koglbauer et al. (2011) developed an anticipative training concept for recovery from unusual attitudes, stalls, and spins that was based on the anticipation-action-comparison model (Kallus et al., 1997). The reader is referred to FlightSimTUGraz (2012) for a video demonstration of the recovery maneuvers in real aircraft. In developing the training concept, they analyzed expert performance (Boucsein et al., 2011), reviewed state-of-the-art recovery procedures (Love, 1996; Stowell, 1999), and verified the concept in pre-tests conducted with novice pilots.

Interestingly, a novice pilot reported how startling the first experience of such upset maneuvers and spins can be. The trainee's mental picture included elements of an upside-down environment, unusual rotations and accelerations combined with unusual g-strain signals of one's own body, high emotional arousal, and high perceived time pressure for applying recovery actions. Flying inverted or with excessive pitch attitude can disturb the sense of control and comfort of a pilot used to flying straight-and-level. For this novice pilot, it was difficult to identify the memorized triggers, to remember the procedure, and to focus on the action effects. The instructor had valuable contributions in helping the trainee to focus on actions and effects. Assisting trainees to focus on critical elements is an important contribution to their construction of correct representations of unusual flight situations. Also, the timely contribution of the instructor in connecting situational pictures to recovery actions is essential for creating the correct action-effect models. Trainees also need time to develop appropriate higher-order mental models, that is, to filter the overwhelming information and detect and store the relevant and essential patterns of information.

For inclusion in the anticipation-based training concept, the recovery actions of an expert pilot were modelled into anticipation–action–comparison units (Koglbauer et al., 2011). The sequences of triggers, goals, and action–effect relationships were transposed in written briefings containing pictures of triggers, action–effects, and memory items for the action–effects (e.g., power, push, roll, recovered). Figure 4.3 illustrates one of these briefings, the anticipation-based briefing for the recovery of an overbanked attitude characterized by a bank angle of 150 degrees and 5 degrees nose down. Recovery actions were: Reduce power to idle, push the elevator to stop the nose from dropping, and roll the shortest way upright. By easily pulling the nose to the horizon, the aircraft is brought back to level flight. After that power is applied smoothly. The wording "power–push–roll" has been adopted from Stowell (1999) and changed to "power–push–roll–recovered." The trainees were briefed on possible errors such as keeping full power, trying to pull a split S, excessive pull of the control stick on recovery, or rolling the long way.

The recovery procedure as illustrated in Figure 4.3 was presented in similar written briefings for all studied maneuvers. In addition, the trainees received a verbal briefing with the instructor on the ground, followed by an in-flight demonstration of maneuvers by the instructor and a first in-flight test of the pilot's ability to apply the procedure. Thus, the pilots could learn the real sensations of motion, could identify visual cues for aircraft rotations (pitch, yaw and roll), and could probe action–effect–units. After the real flight, the pilots trained in a fixed-base simulator with sufficient visual fidelity to practice the tasks, using the anticipation-based briefing. On a subsequent day, the pilots attended a simulator test and a post-test in the aircraft.

The anticipation-based training concept was tested with 33 pilots assigned to an experimental and a control group. Results showed significant effects of the anticipation-based training on pilots' performance, workload, emotion, psychophysiological activation, and a transfer of skills from simulator to real flight (Koglbauer et al., 2011). In addition, the results showed that processes of anticipation, preparation, action, and comparison could be objectively identified in psychophysiological indicators of different types of psychophysiological arousal, as described by Boucsein and Backs (2009). Physiological data were analyzed for three different phases of each flight maneuver: anticipation, aircraft recovery, and post-recovery. For example, the experimental group had lower NS.SCR frequency than the control group, an effect that was already visible during the anticipative phase, as illustrated

Safety goal: Recovery to straight and level flight, as quick as possible

Upset attitude: Roll angle of 150 degrees left, cruise power and 5 degrees pitch down

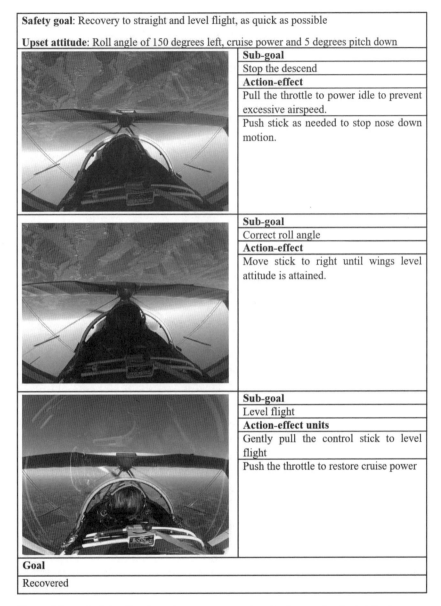

	Sub-goal
	Stop the descend
	Action-effect
	Pull the throttle to power idle to prevent excessive airspeed.
	Push stick as needed to stop nose down motion.
	Sub-goal
	Correct roll angle
	Action-effect
	Move stick to right until wings level attitude is attained.
	Sub-goal
	Level flight
	Action-effect units
	Gently pull the control stick to level flight
	Push the throttle to restore cruise power

Goal
Recovered

Figure 4.3   Anticipation-based recovery procedure for the overbanked attitude.

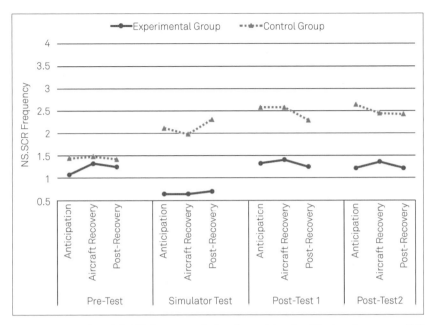

Figure 4.4   Mean NS.SCR frequency during the anticipation (A), aircraft recovery (AR) and post-recovery phases across all maneuvers. From Koglbauer, 2009.

in Figure 4.4 (Koglbauer, 2009). In accordance with Boucsein and Backs (2009), lower NS.SCR frequency indicates lower affect arousal.

In summary, these studies show applications of the anticipatory processing paradigm on pilot training. Anticipation-based training methods assist trainees in developing correct mental models by highlighting goals and sub-goals, action–effect relationships, and essential cues, and by providing specific feedback to adjust anticipations (e.g., time to collision). Similarly, feedback is an essential mechanism in the formation of action–effect relationships and internal models of action.

Applications of the Anticipatory Paradigm to Cockpit Engineering

Besides training, cockpit engineering can support the anticipatory performance of a pilot. Parasuraman et al. (2000) classified different *types* of automation in terms of human information processing: Sensory processing, perception, working memory, decision- making, and response selection. Within types of automation, different *levels* of automation may be applied including decision and action (Parasuraman et al., 2000). At the highest level the automation decides and acts, without any control inputs by the human operator. At the lowest level all decisions and actions are allocated to the human.

For example, in commercial aviation, pilots use an automated traffic alert and collision avoidance system (TCAS) that informs the pilot about traffic in the vicinity, warns about imminent collision, indicates an avoidance action, and notifies when the pilot is clear of traffic (Federal Aviation Administration, 2014). Traffic displays to support pilots' anticipative processes in collision threat detection and avoidance have been the subject of research (Haberkorn et al., 2013; Haberkorn et al., 2014; Van Dam et al., 2008; Wickens et al., 2000). Wickens et al. (2000) developed a *"predictive track"* that was displayed with and without a *"threat vector"* indicating the relative approach angle of a conflicting aircraft. Simulator tests showed that pilots spent significantly less time engaged in conflicts when using the predictive track with the threat vector, but their subjective workload was not reduced.

Van Dam et al. (2008) used the ecological interface approach (Vicente & Rasmussen, 1992) to design the state vector envelope display (XATP) that shows a complex forward view of the conflict situation including *"forbidden zones"* that must be avoided by the pilot in order to avoid an imminent collision. Simulator tests showed that the XATP improved conflict awareness and the estimation of the conflict's geometry and urgency in airline pilots.

Haberkorn et al. (2013) investigated pilots' reactions to a TCAS-like display during VFR flight. In particular types of airspace, in VFR flight, pilots are responsible to see-and-avoid other air vehicles by scanning the scenery outside the window. Haberkorn et al. (2013) identified multiple issues encountered by pilots using a TCAS-like traffic display in simulated flight. TCAS was designed to generate avoidance actions in instrument flight rules (IFR) flight and was shown to provide only a limited part of the information needed to avoid collisions in VFR flight. On the basis of an analysis of conflict information needed by VFR pilots, Haberkorn et al. (2014) subsequently developed traffic displays that combined multiple predictive features such as traffic position and orientation, vehicle type, and absolute, relative, and priority tracks (Figure 4.5). Because the type of air vehicle determines the priority in VFR flight, this was considered an essential cue. The display variants were evaluated by 21 pilots in simulated conflict scenarios. The display variant that combined oriented air vehicle symbols and the relative track (Figure 4.5d), and the variant showing the priority cue (Figure 4.5e) were appreciated as being the most preferred designs. These variants also supported the pilots in taking significantly faster conflict decisions with lower mental demand as compared with the display of conventional and oriented air vehicle symbols (Figure 4.5b), the absolute track (Figure 4.5c), or the TCAS-like symbols (Figure 4.5a).

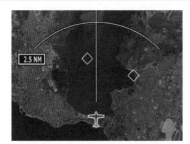
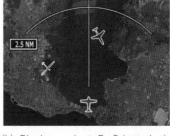

(a) Display variant A: The baseline display. Diamond shapes denote positions of intruding air vehicles. The ownship is depicted by a light aircraft symbol.

(b) Display variant B: Oriented air vehicle symbols denote positions and direction of intruding air vehicles (here: glider from left, small jet ahead).

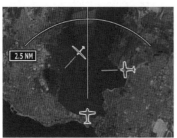
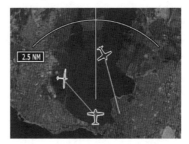

(c) Display variant C: Oriented aircraft symbols with 'absolute' trackline denote positions and directions of intruding air vehicles (here: glider ahead, light aircraft from right).

(d) Display variant D: Oriented aircraft symbols with relative trackline (here: glider from left on a predicted collision course with the ownship, light aircraft ahead). The relative line shows if traffic is on collision course or not.

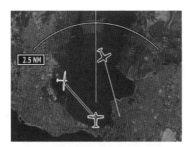

(e) Display variant E: Oriented aircraft symbols with relative track & priority line (here: glider from left has priority, light aircraft ahead).

Figure 4.5   Display variants with anticipative cues. Reprinted with permission from "Traffic Displays for Visual Flight Indicating Track and Priority Cues" by T. Haberkorn, I. Koglbauer, and R. Braunstingl, 2014, *IEEE Transactions on Human-Machine Systems, 44*(6), p. 760. © 2014 IEEE.

These studies show that cockpit automation can support pilots' anticipatory performance. The next section addresses predictive automation in air traffic management (ATM).

Applications of the Anticipatory Paradigm to ATM Systems

ATM relies on a collaborative and automated concept of operations that requires shared situational awareness of the stakeholders. Strategic air traffic control is supported by a number of predictive tools, such as trajectory prediction and conflict detection and resolution tools that, in order to be effective, should match the concept of operations as close as possible (Schuster & Ochieng, 2014).

Kearney et al. (2016) redesigned a short-term conflict alert (STCA) to better match the context of operations. They designed a semantic alert similar to TCAS and compared it with the conventional beep-tone alert. Tests were conducted with 26 air traffic control officers (ATCOs) in the training simulator at the Irish Aviation Authority (Kearney et al., 2016). The semantic alert resulted in a specific eye-movement pattern in ATCOs characterized by shorter saccade duration, higher saccade velocity, and more and longer fixations on the displayed conflict as compared with the beep-tone. Thus, Kearney et al. (2016) showed that alert design significantly improves ATCOs' situational awareness and the time needed for conflict resolution.

Potential Applications to Multiple Remote Tower Design and Operations

Research on remote tower operations has flourished in the past two decades and has become a strategic research topic in both Europe and the United States. Currently, in a "*remote tower*" ATCOs can control traffic at an aerodrome from a distant virtual control "*tower*" using special equipment. Thus, in a remote tower ATCOs' anticipatory processing relies completely on the equipment used for gathering information, feedback, and executing air traffic control by means of verbal communication.

Kearney and Li (2018) addressed ATCOs' cognitive processing in simultaneous control of traffic at multiple remote towers. The remote tower included an out the window visualization (OTW), electronic flight strip (EFS) system, a voice communication system (TEL), and radar data processing

(RDP). During live test trials one ATCO located in Dublin, Ireland, controlled traffic at both Cork and Shannon airports. A total of three ATCOs holding multiple ratings participated in the experiment. Kearney and Li (2018) assessed ATCOs' cognitive processing based on their eye movements across four areas of interests: RDP, EFS, TEL, and OTW. They found that the ATCOs' number of fixations on RDP was significantly larger than on EFS and TEL, but was similar to the fixations count on OTW. The saccade amplitude was significantly larger for OTW as compared with RDP, EFS, and TEL. ATCOs' long fixations on RDP and OTW, and the workload induced by using TEL, were identified as the biggest challenge of single-ATCO operation of multiple remote towers (Kearney & Li, 2018). Kearney and Li (2018) recommended an adjustment of the equipment to the specific context of operations and multiple roles in further research.

In terms of the anticipatory paradigm, these results from Kearney and Li (2018) can be interpreted as a mismatch between ATCOs' anticipated traffic picture and the picture displayed on the OTW. The OTW mapped a 360-degrees view of the selected airport and its surroundings into 208-degrees panoramic visualization. The ATCOs' mental model might have been based on the 360-degree field of sight from the real towers, resulting in a mismatch between the anticipated and real mental pictures, and the anticipated and real effects. For further development of the technology supporting multiple remote towers operations, the anticipatory processing paradigm could be applied to determining and displaying critical pictures, goal representations, and action models. In addition, the anticipatory paradigm could be applied to the design of training and conversion training for ATCOs working in multiple remote towers.

Application to Artificial Intelligence

Artificial intelligence (AI) has been successfully designed and tested in aviation. In a widely medialized competition, AI recently won all five dogfights against a human US Air Force pilot (Wolf, 2020). AI uses knowledge of learning and cognition for building intelligent agents (Poole & Mackworth, 2017). Anticipatory learning mechanisms have been validated with computational models used in robots (Borisov & Vasilyev, 2002; Demiris, 2007) and predictive vehicle control algorithms (Dollar & Vahidi, 2018). Butz (2016) proposed a "unifying, sub-symbolic, computational theory of cognition" based on the anticipatory behavioral control paradigm, AI and machine learning theories, reinforcement learning, generative artificial neural networks, and other concepts. Butz's (2016) theory sees behavior, attention, and thought as being anticipatory. The brain is seen as a predictive encoding system in which episodes are perceived, imagined, or remembered and event schema-encodings predict how a scenario may change over time (Butz, 2016). On the basis of his theory, Butz (2016) proposed an artificial self-developing system that has sensory and motor capabilities and motivation to be released into "any available, sufficiently rich virtual reality simulation." In his view, future research of the cognitive development of AI is a major step forward in understanding both human and artificial cognition. While the interest in AI is growing, it is important to understand ethical implications and safety risks, given that such self-developing, artificial, cognitive creatures should not exceed sociotechnical control capabilities. Currently, the "Ethics Guidelines for Trustworthy Artificial Intelligence (AI)" (European Commission, 2019) apply in Europe.

Conclusion

Anticipatory behavioral control is essential for effective human performance in aviation, and can be fostered by training and equipment design. Anticipation-based training methods assist trainees in developing correct mental models, goal representations, and action–effect models by highlighting essential cues, providing feedback, and assisting with match -comparisons to better adjust anticipations. In addition, engineered systems providing anticipative cues (e.g., predictive automation) have a significant impact on improving human cognition and performance, providing that they match the context of operation and task requirements. Computational anticipatory agents have been developed and tested in the past few decades. The anticipatory behavioral control paradigm is a core element with high potential for the future development of AI in aviation.

References

Borisov, A., & Vasilyev, A. (2002). Learning classifier systems in autonomous agent control tasks. In M. Malkowskiy & K. Varov (Eds.), *Proceedings of the Fifth International Conference on Application of Fuzzy Systems and Soft Computing* (pp. 36–42). Milan, Italy. https://doi.org/10.1.1.103.966&rep=rep1&type=pdf

Boucsein, W., & Backs, W. (2009). The psychophysiology of emotion, arousal, and personality: methods and models. In V. G. Duffy (Ed.) *Handbook of digital human modeling. Research for applied ergonomics and human factors engineering* (pp. 35-1/35-8). CRC Press, Taylor & Francis.

Boucsein, W., Koglbauer, I., Braunstingl, R., & Kallus, K. W. (2011). The use of psychophysiological measures during complex flight manoeuvers – an expert pilot study. In J. H. Westerink, M. Krans, & M. Ouwererk (Eds.), *Sensing emotions. The impact of con-*

text on experience measurements (pp. 53‒63). Springer. https://doi.org/10.1007/978-90-481-3258-4_4

Butz, M. V. (2016). Toward a unified sub-symbolic computational theory of cognition. *Frontiers in Psychology, 7*, 925. https://doi.org/10.3389/fpsyg.2016.00925

Demiris, Y. (2007). Prediction of intent in robotics and multi-agent systems. *Cognitive Processing, 8*, 151‒158. https://doi.org/10.1007/s10339-007-0168-9

Dollar, R. A., & Vahidi, A. (2018). Efficient and collision-free anticipative cruise control in randomly mixed strings. *IEEE Transactions on Intelligent Vehicles, 3*(4), 439‒452. https://doi.org/10.1109/TIV.2018.2873895

Endsley, M. R. (1988). Design and evaluation for situation awareness enhancement. In HFES (Ed.), *Proceedings of the Human Factors Society 32nd Annual Meeting* (pp. 97‒101). Human Factors and Ergonomics Society. https://doi.org/10.1177/154193128803200221

Endsley, M. R. (2000). Theoretical underpinnings of situation awareness: A critical review. In M. R. Endsley, & D. J. Garland (Eds.), *Situation awareness analysis and measurement* (pp. 3‒32). Lawrence Erlbaum Associates. https://doi.org/10.1201/b12461

European Commission. (2019). *Ethics guidelines for trustworthy artificial intelligence (AI)*. https://ec.europa.eu/futurium/en/ai-alliance-consultation/guidelines#Top

Federal Aviation Administration. (2014). *Introduction to TCAS II Version 7.1*. http://www.skybrary.aero/bookshelf/books/1927.pdf

FlightSimTUGraz. (2012). *Emergency recovery* [Video]. https://www.youtube.com/watch?v=xaPo4UCTBCQ

Haberkorn, T., Koglbauer, I., & Braunstingl, R. (2014). Traffic displays for visual flight indicating track and priority cues. *IEEE Transactions on Human-Machine Systems, 44*(6), 755‒766. https://doi.org/10.1109/THMS.2014.2352496

Haberkorn, T., Koglbauer, I., Braunstingl, R., & Prehofer, B. (2013). Requirements for future collision avoidance systems in visual flight: a human-centered approach. *IEEE Transactions on Human-Machine Systems, 43*(6), 583‒594. https://doi.org/10.1109/THMS.2013.2284784

Hoffmann, J. (1993). *Vorhersage und Erkenntnis. Die Funktion von Antizipationen in der menschlichen Verhaltenssteuerung und Wahrnehmung* [The function of anticipations in human behavioral control and perception]. Hogrefe.

Hoffmann, J. (2003). Anticipatory behavioral control. In M. V. Butz, O. Sigaud & P. Gerard (Eds.), *Anticipatory behaviour in adaptive learning systems* (pp. 44‒65). Springer. https://doi.org/10.1007/978-3-540-45002-3_4

Kallus, K. W. (2009). Situationsbewusstsein und antizipative Prozesse [Situational awareness and anticipatory processes]. *Zeitschrift für Arbeitswissenschaft: Zentralblatt für Arbeitswissenschaft und soziale Betriebspraxis, 63*(1), 17‒22.

Kallus, K. W. (2012). Anticipatory processes in critical flight situations. In A. de Voogt, & T. D'Oliveira (Eds.), *Mechanisms in the chain of safety. Research and operational experiences in aviation psychology* (pp. 97‒106). Ashgate Publishing Ltd.

Kallus, K. W., Barbarino, M., & van Damme, V. (1997). *Model of the cognitive aspects of air traffic control*. (Report No. HUM.ET1.ST01.1000-REP-02). EUROCONTROL.

Kallus, K. W., & Tropper, K. (2007). Anticipatory processes in critical flight situations. In ISAP (Ed.), *Proceedings of the International Symposium on Aviation Psychology* (pp. 309‒314). Wright State University. https://corescholar.libraries.wright.edu/isap_2007/82

Kearney, P., Li, W. C., & Lin, J. J. H. (2016). The impact of alerting design on air traffic controllers' response to conflict detection and resolution. *International Journal of Industrial Ergonomics, 56*, 51–58. https://doi.org/10.1016/j.ergon.2016.09.002

Kearney, P., & Li, W. C. (2018). Multiple remote tower for Single European Sky: The evolution from initial operational concept to regulatory approved implementation. *Transportation Research Part A, 116*, 15–30. https://doi.org/10.1016/j.tra.2018.06.005

Koglbauer, I. (2009). *Multidimensional approach of threat and error management training for VFR pilots: Evaluation of anticipative training effects during simulated and real flight.* (Unpublished doctoral dissertation). Karl Franzens University of Graz, Austria.

Koglbauer, I. (2015a). Simulator training improves the estimation of collision parameters and the performance of student pilots. *Procedia – Social and Behavioral Sciences, 209*, 261–267. https://doi.org/10.1016/j.sbspro.2015.11.231

Koglbauer, I. (2015b). Gender differences in time perception. In R. Hoffman, P. A. Hancock, M. Scerbo, R. Parasuraman, & J. L. Szalma (Eds.), *The Cambridge handbook of applied perception research* (pp. 1004–1028). Cambridge University Press. https://doi.org/10.1017/CBO9780511973017.059

Koglbauer, I., & Braunstingl, R. (2018). Ab initio pilot training for traffic separation and visual airport procedures in a naturalistic flight simulation environment. *Transportation Research Part F: Psychology and Behavior, 58*, 1–10. https://doi.org/10.1016/j.trf.2018.05.023

Koglbauer, I., Kallus, K. W., Braunstingl, R., & Boucsein, W. (2011). Recovery training in simulator improves performance and psychophysiological state of pilots during simulated and real visual flight rules flight. *International Journal of Aviation Psychology, 21*(4), 307–324. https://doi.org/10.1080/10508414.2011.606741

Kunde, W., Kiesel, A., & Hoffmann, J. (2003). Conscious control over the content of unconscious cognition. *Cognition, 88*, 223–242. https://doi.org/10.1016/S0010-0277(03)00023-4

Love, M. C. (1996). *Spin management and recovery.* Mc Graw Hill.

Parasuraman, R., Sheridan, T. B., & Wickens, C. D. (2000). A model for types and levels of human interaction with automation. *IEEE Transactions on Systems, Man Cybernetics, Part A, 30*(3), 286–297. https://doi.org/10.1109/3468.844354

Poole, D. L., & Mackworth, A. K. (2017). *Artificial intelligence: Foundations of computational agents* (2nd ed.). Cambridge University Press. https://doi.org/10.1017/9781108164085

Schuster, W., & Ochieng, W. (2014). Performance requirements of future trajectory prediction and conflict detection and resolution tools within SESAR and NextGen: Framework for the derivation and discussion. *Journal of Air Transport Management, 35*, 92–101. https://doi.org/10.1016/j.jairtraman.2013.11.005

Stowell, R. (1999). *Innovations in stall/spin awareness training.* Second Annual Instructor Conference, Embry-Riddle Aeronautical University, Daytona Beach, Florida.

Talker, C. M., & Kallus, K. (2015). Anticipatorily controlled top-down processes influence the impact of Coriolis effects. In Wright State University (Ed.), *Proceedings of the 18th International Symposium on Aviation Psychology* (pp. 207–212). ISAP. https://corescholar.libraries.wright.edu/isap_2015/72

Van Dam, S. B. J., Steens, C. L. A., Mulder, M., & Van Paassen, M. M. (2008). Evaluation of two pilot self-separation displays using conflict situation measurements. In IEEE (Ed.), *Proceedings of the IEEE International Conference on Systems, Man and Cybernetics* (pp. 3558–3563). IEEE. https://doi.org/10.1109/ICSMC.2008.4811850

Vicente, K. J., & Rasmussen, J. (1992). Ecological interface design: Theoretical foundations. *IEEE Transactions on Systems, Man and Cybernetics, 22*(4), 589–606. https://doi.org/10.1109/21.156574

Wickens, C. D., Gempler, K., & Morphew, M. E. (2000). Workload and reliability of predictor displays in aircraft traffic avoidance. *Transportation Human Factors, 2*(2), 99–126. https://doi.org/10.1207/STHF0202_01

Wolfe, F. (2020, September). Heron systems shows future potential of AI in win over top F-16 weapons instructor. *Aviation Today.* https://www.aviationtoday.com/2020/08/24/heron-systems-shows-future-potential-ai-win-top-f-16-weapons-instructor/

Chapter 5
Research Methods for Understanding Spatial Disorientation in Pilots

Eric Groen

Abstract

Spatial disorientation (SD) can be greatly confusing to pilots and impact their performance, potentially with catastrophic results, which makes it a relevant research topic for aviation psychologists. Due to its multifaceted nature, SD can be investigated by means of a variety of research methods. The choice of the adequate method depends on the research question at hand. For example, since SD is a direct result of inaccurate perception of aircraft motions, research can be aimed at unraveling its neurophysiological mechanisms. This may involve psychophysical methods derived from vestibular or visual sciences. Research can also focus on the effect of fatigue, or workload, on a pilot's susceptibility to SD, using pilot state monitoring techniques, such as gaze tracking. Yet other research areas involve the development of effective countermeasures against SD in-flight, or simulator scenarios for SD awareness training on the ground. The challenge with the latter is to generate realistic motion cues, while avoiding false cues. As a final example, SD research can involve the investigation of flight safety events, which can benefit from human perception models. In short, SD research can be aimed at improving: (1) knowledge about the etiology of SD; (2) anti-disorientation training in simulators or aircraft; (3) incident and accident analysis. This chapter provides an overview of commonly applied research methods in SD research, with attention to their advantages as well as limitations.

Keywords: perception, sensory physiology, vestibular, visual, illusions, startle, simulation

Introduction

Spatial disorientation (SD) in-flight is known as an erroneous perception of the motion or attitude of the aircraft, and is primarily caused by misleading sensory information. Aircraft motions, sensed by the vestibular system in the inner ear, can be unreliable because they either remain under the perception threshold or provide ambiguous cues. But, also visual cues in the outside environment can be deceptive, such as a false horizon caused by a sloping cloud deck. The chance that unreliable sensory information develops into SD depends on other factors, such as distraction, fatigue, or high workload. Obviously, SD can have serious consequences for flight safety, especially when the pilot is unaware of being disoriented. The latter situation, designated Type-I disorientation, can trigger incorrect control inputs and, in the worst case, lead to controlled flight into terrain (CFIT). Another possibility is that pilots suddenly realize a mismatch between their sensations and the information shown on the instruments. This so-called Type-II disorientation can be very confusing, and even cause a startle response, which may impair one's ability to understand what is going on (Type-III disorientation). In most cases, however, pilots manage to avoid or recognize disorientation in a timely way by good flight preparation, regularly checking the flight instruments, and by adequate crew coordination.

Because SD covers so many human factor aspects it is an interesting research topic for scientists from various disciplines, including visual and vestibular perception, aviation psychology, aerospace medicine, human physiology, simulator engineering, and accident investigation. Clearly, this chapter cannot describe all the possible methods that can be applied in the area of SD. Instead, the most relevant "ingredients" for SD research will be discussed. The first sections deal with different ways to generate an SD stimulus, followed by several sections on a pilot's responses to SD stimuli. The text also includes example studies to illustrate how these topics have been investigated previously.

Vestibular Stimulus

The vestibular system in the inner ear consists of two functionally different sensors: the semicircular canals and the otolith organs, which respond to angular and linear motions of the head, respectively (Guedry, 1974). Usually, vestibular stimuli are expressed in head-centered coordinates, as depicted in Figure 5.1. The effective stimulus for the semicircular canals consists of angular acceleration (deg/s^2), although in the frequency range of natural head movements (roughly 0.1–5 Hz) we perceive angular rate (deg/s). The stimulus for the otolith organs consists of linear accelerations (m/s^2), caused by inertial motion (translation) of the head, as well as tilt relative to gravity (the gravitational acceleration). Hence, the

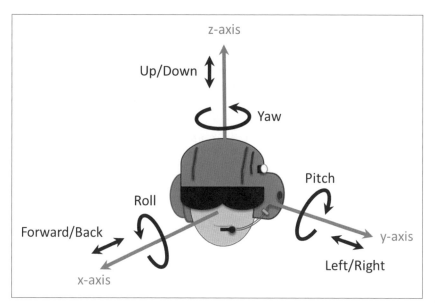

Figure 5.1   Head-centered coordinate system used to indicate angular and linear self-motion in the sagittal, or x-axis; transversal, or y-axis; and longitudinal, or z-axis.

input is the vector sum of all linear accelerations: designated the gravito-inertial acceleration (GIA). Sometimes the GIA is also referred to as "specific force."

Aircraft motions can be disorienting because they produce different vestibular stimulus patterns than natural head movements. Some aircraft motions remain below the perception threshold (e.g., undetected drift), whereas others induce noticeable but ambiguous sensations. Ambiguities in the perception of angular motion arise from the semicircular canals being insensitive to slowly changing or constant rate turns. This characteristic is responsible for *somatogyral illusions*, such as the *post-roll illusion* (Ercoline et al., 2000; Nooij & Groen, 2011) and the *graveyard spin* (Previc & Ercoline, 2004). Furthermore, head movements during an ongoing turn result in cross-coupled stimulation of the semicircular canals, which cause the Coriolis illusion: a false sensation of a change in aircraft pitch or roll, depending on the directions of the head movement and the turn (Collins, 1968; Guedry & Benson, 1978). Another category of SD, the *somatogravic illusions*, arise from perceptual ambiguities of the specific force: a linear acceleration causes a reorientation of the specific force in head coordinates, similar to the reorientation of gravity during tilt of the head. Without additional visual references, forward acceleration of an aircraft can thus be misperceived as pitching up. For more background information on the vestibular mechanisms of SD, the reader is referred to Previc and Ercoline (2004) and Stott (2013).

In reporting vestibular experiments, it is important to clearly specify the motion stimulus as well as the orientation (attitude) of the participant (aircraft) relative to gravity. Considering the characteristics of the vestibular system, angular rates (preferably also accelerations) and linear accelerations (specific force) are most interesting, measured at the position of the pilot's head. The displacement, or angle, is less relevant because humans do not accurately perceive these dimensions, also under normal conditions.

Visual Stimulus

In clear daylight, our natural environment provides useful visual cues to guide our self-motion and orientation. We can judge our self-motion from the optic flow of the environment on our retina, and our orientation from visual features that define up. In good visibility, visual cues help pilots judge the aircraft's attitude and to disambiguate vestibular cues that may otherwise lead to SD. For example, Tokumaru et al. (1998) showed that the presence of a visible horizon in the outside visual significantly reduced the magnitude of the somatogravic illusion measured in a centrifuge-based simulator. Interestingly, according to an earlier study, a horizon presented inside a helmet-mounted display (HMD) did not successfully suppress the somatogravic illusion (Previc et al. 1992). The authors speculate that this was due to the poor resolution of the HMD. Current HMDs are probably more effective as they offer more realism.

In poor visibility, such as fog or night, the lack of visual references may increase the risk of vestibular SD. In other conditions, the visual environment can be disorienting by itself. For example, a sloping cloud deck may erroneously be perceived as the horizon, and a pilot may be tempted to align the aircraft with this *false horizon*. Another example of a disorientating visual condition is a helicopter *brownout* landing, where the rotor downwash causes circulation of dust particles around the cockpit. The dust cloud not only reduces the crew's visibility, but it may also cause (upward) optic flow that induces a false sensation of (downward) motion. Most people are familiar with this kind of illusory self-motion from looking out the window of a stationary train, and seeing the neighboring train depart. Such visually induced sensation of self-motion is known as "vection" (Melcher & Henn, 1981). Conversely, the lack of vection when flying over featureless terrain, such as a smooth water surface, can lead to an underestimation of speed as well as difficulties in judging the altitude. This explains why an approach to an illuminated runway in otherwise dark surroundings, a so-called dark hole approach, can be very challenging to pilots.

Laboratory Devices

The most commonly used motion device for vestibular research is a servo-controlled rotating chair. Rotation devices are useful for investigating the characteristics of the semicircular canals, such as the decay of the after-sensation upon the end of a prolonged turn. A typical stimulus profile has a trapezoid shape, consisting of a steep onset to a certain angular velocity (e.g., 60 deg/s), which is kept constant for a certain period (e.g., 30 s) before being decelerated to a stop. The vestibular response can be measured subjectively (e.g., verbal report of the perceived rotation) or objectively (reflexive eye movements, or *nystagmus*). A rotation chair is also adequate for inducing a Coriolis illusion, by asking (blindfolded) participants to tilt their head during an ongoing body rotation. As the Coriolis sensation can be highly nauseating, it is recommended to limit the number and duration of trials.

A few authors describe the use of galvanic vestibular stimulation (GVS) as an alternative way to induce vestibular stimuli (Malcik 1968; Moore et al., 2011). This technique produces vestibular sensations by applying current directly to the vestibular nerve through electrodes behind the ears. Moore et al. (2011) used bilateral bipolar GVS with 11 pilots while they performed manual landings in a Space Shuttle simulator. The GVS stimuli consisted of a sinusoidal current waveform, with dominant frequencies of 0.16, 0.33, 0.43, and 0.61 Hz, and a maximum current of ± 5 mA, which induced sensations of rocking from side to side. The results showed that the percentage of crash landings increased from 2.3 % without GVS to 9 % with GVS. The number of landings with unacceptable high touchdown speed (> 214 kn) almost doubled with GVS. The authors conclude that GVS is an effective analogue of decrements observed in postflight Shuttle pilot performance.

Visually induced SD can also be investigated in the laboratory by using a moving or tilted visual field. Some classic studies on vection were performed with an optokinetic drum, that is, a rotatable cylinder decorated with vertical stripes (Dichgans & Brandt, 1978). Other studies used a displaced visual field (Asch & Witkin, 1948), or a tilting room to determine the role of visual cues on orientation perception (Allison et al., 1999; Howard & Childerson, 1994). Figure 5.2 shows a combination of a visual stimulus and rotating chair to study certain visual–vestibular interactions. Today's virtual reality (VR) technologies offer great flexibility in generating all kinds of visual stimuli, although there may be limitations in terms of spatiotemporal resolution and field of view.

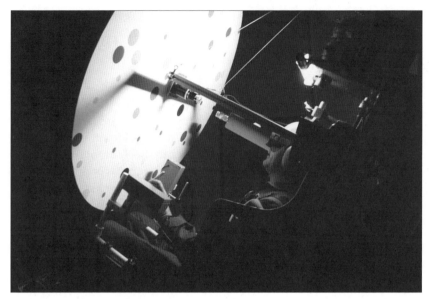

Figure 5.2   Experimental set-up in a rotating chair to investigate the interaction between vestibular cues on body tilt with a visually induced sensation of
roll motion (vection) in a rotating chair. The perceived vection magnitude
is indicated by means of a joystick. Reprinted with permission from Netherlands Organization for Applied Scientific Research (Nederlandse Organisatie voor Toegepast Natuurwetenschappelijk Onderzoek – TNO).
© TNO.

Although laboratory devices usually have only one or two degrees of freedom (DoF), their great advantage is that the motion stimulus can be controlled with great precision and reproducibility. Because the stimulus is ex-
actly known, there is a clear relation with the participant's response. This is
useful for the determination of a stimulus–response relationship for a wide
range of stimulus frequencies. Another advantage of laboratory devices is
that they normally have low operational costs compared with flight simulators or real aircraft.

Limitations of Laboratory Devices

One of the main limitations of laboratory devices is that, despite their con-
trollability, the motion stimulus is extremely simplified compared with motions in real flight. For example, due to the forward location of the cockpit
in large aircraft, rotations (yaw or pitch) also produce parasitical linear
accelerations (sway or heave, respectively) at the level of the pilot's head,

which cannot be reproduced on a rotating chair. In addition, rotating chairs lack the capability to generate sustained G-loads, except for eccentric devices with a small arm (<1 m) that enable small centripetal accelerations. Another limitation is that laboratory devices normally do not feature a cockpit environment and lack items such as cockpit instruments, flight controls, and out-the-window visual scenery. However, VR technologies eliminate some of these limitations, and make it possible to immerse someone in a visual (cockpit) environment without the need of an advanced projection system.

Ground-Based Simulator

Flight simulators enable pilots to perform a flight task in a representative environment, including flight controls, instruments, and out-the-window (OTW) scenery. Theoretically, visual SD illusions can be investigated in a fixed-base simulator, consisting of a non-moving cockpit and an OTW visual display. However, for actively piloted scenarios a moving-base simulator is preferred, because it enhances the feel of flying. Obviously, the generation of vestibular SD effects requires a motion platform (Kallus et al., 2011). The most widely used motion platform in full flight simulation is the hexapod type. Its six linear actuators are controlled by the simulator's motion driving algorithms, or *washout filters*, which convert the aircraft motions from the flight model into simulator platform motion. Because of the limited stroke length of the actuators, motion cues are usually being washed out (hence the name "washout filter"), primarily reproducing the accelerations, or *onset* cues. Usually, the sustained longitudinal acceleration during takeoff is simulated by the backward pitch of the simulator (Groen & Bles, 2004; Groen et al., 2001). Although a hexapod-type platform has limited capabilities to induce vestibular illusions, some illusions may be "cheated." For example, Klyde et al. (2016) used excessive platform pitch to mimic the sensation of a somatogravic illusion during a go-around.

Special Devices

As an alternative to the hexapod platform, various manufacturers have developed special-purpose motion devices to reproduce vestibular SD effects. So-called spinning devices have an additional turn table (to induce somatogyral illusions), and *G-devices* have a centrifuge capability to induce sustained G-loads. A combination of a spinning and G-device is the DESDEMONA simulator (Figure 5.3) with a gimbaled cockpit for unlimited three-dimensional (3-D) rotations, an 8-m horizontal and 2-m vertical drive for linear motions (e.g., helicopter hover), and a 4-m centrifuge arm for G-loads up to 3 g (Bles & Groen, 2009; Correia et al., 2013; Ledegang & Groen, 2015).

The investigation of the somatogravic illusion can be done in a human centrifuge with a capability of *G-pointing*, so that the gondola can be oriented in such a way that the G-load is constantly aligned with the pilot's x-axis. This differs from high-G training, where the G-load is oriented along the pilot's longitudinal, or z-axis, to practice the *anti-G straining maneuver*. For example, Cohen et al. (1973) and Cohen (1976) investigated the somatogravic illusion by reproducing the G-profile of a 4-g catapult launch by a quick rotation of the centrifuge over 180 deg in 3.2 s, while simultaneously rotating the gondola over 360 deg in yaw, so that the G-load was always front-to-back. The participants' task was to adjust the height of a target light projected on a screen in front of them so that it appeared at eye level. The results showed that the G-stimulus induced a 10-deg elevation of perceived eye level (oculogravic illusion). When the participants were given active control of the cabin's orientation, they pitched it down by about 10 deg, indicating a somatogravic illusion.

Because the main purpose of SD devices is to demonstrate the effects of SD, rather than to teach how to fly the aircraft, they normally feature a ge-

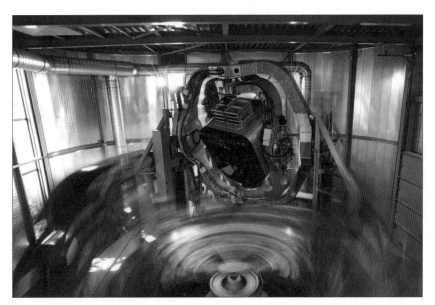

Figure 5.3   The DESDEMONA centrifuge-based research simulator. Reprinted with permission from TNO. © TNO.

neric cockpit, representative of some kind of aircraft (e.g., trainer, fighter, or helicopter). The same applies to the flight model. Many of these devices have preprogrammed SD scenarios, which can be inserted into a flight scenario to investigate their effects on pilot behavior (Ledegang & Groen, 2018; Previc et al., 2007, 2009).

Limitations of Simulators

In most cases, simulator motion is only an approximation of the real aircraft, and may be compromised by *false cues*. In general, simulator fidelity suffers more from false cues than it gains from correct cues and should be avoided as much as possible (Groen et al., 2001). Sometimes it may be possible to adapt the motion cueing to reduce false cues (Groen et al., 2007), but when this is not possible it should be considered to investigate a different maneuver.

In contrast to research simulators such as DESDEMONA, it may be difficult to change the motion settings of a commercial device without the help of the manufacturer. The same is true for the extraction of data from the device (e.g., aircraft motions, platform motion, flight parameters, and control inputs). Investigators may need to collect their own data, for example, by means of an inertial measurement unit on the cabin floor. Special care is needed to synchronize the measurement equipment with the simulation for post hoc analysis of the data. Simulators may also have higher operating costs than laboratory devices. Finally, one should keep in mind that pilots usually know that they will experience some kind of non-normal situation in a simulator, which makes it difficult to mislead or surprise a pilot to the same extent as can occur in real flight.

Aircraft

In-flight SD demonstrations can be very compelling. The obvious advantage of an aircraft is that the stimuli are realistic, without the motion artifacts (false cues, washout) observed in ground-based devices. This is particularly the case for coordinated turns, which cannot be simulated by tilting a motion platform (because this would give a sensation of uncoordinated flight). Apart from realistic motion cues, aircraft also have the possibility to induce a real startle response in pilots, for example, by exposure to an unusual attitude.

As an example of in-flight SD research, McCarthy and Stott (1994) evaluated the inversion illusion in a jet training aircraft. The flight profile started with a longitudinal acceleration of 0.15–0.25 g from 200 to 250 kts in level flight, followed by a gentle pull into a stable 250-kts climb for 30 s, followed by a push to achieve a negative vertical acceleration of –1.0 g for 6 s. The verbal responses of 13 participants were recorded, whose vision was occluded by a black cloth over the visor of the helmet. The paper does not mention any recordings of aircraft motions or vibrations, but given the subjective nature of the responses this does not seem a big problem. The results showed that nine participants perceived sensations of backward rotation and inversion. This sensation can be considered a somatogravic illusion, caused by the backward rotation of the GIA during the maneuver.

In another in-flight study with 40 participants, Landman et al. (2019) showed that SD can trigger roll reversal errors (roll inputs in the undesired direction) when using the attitude indicator (AI). In three different conditions, the test pilot put the aircraft in a roll attitude while the participants were blindfolded, before they were allowed to look at the AI and take control. In the control condition, the maneuver was flown in a normal way so that the participant's sensation matched the roll angle shown on the AI. In two other SD conditions, the maneuver induced a false sensation of roll (the "Leans"), which did not match the angle shown on the AI. In both SD conditions the participants made 60 % of roll reversal errors, compared with 20 % in the control condition. Since all participants in this study were non-pilots, it can be argued that professional pilots will make fewer errors in interpreting the AI. However, other research has shown that even pilots sometimes make roll reversal errors, albeit less frequent than non-pilots (e.g., Beringer et al., 1975). Landman et al. (2019) suggest that pilots may also become more sensitive to misinterpretation of the AI when their own sensation of roll is in conflict with the roll shown on the AI, especially in critical situations with little time to resolve this conflict.

The occurrence of roll reversal errors is particularly interesting given that the AI is the most important cockpit instrument to remain spatially orientated. A possible explanation is that the moving horizon symbol behind a fixed aircraft symbol in the Western-type AI seems to be more confusing than the Eastern-type AI where the aircraft symbol moves in front of a fixed horizon (Müller et al., 2019).

Limitations of In-Flight Studies

In-flight studies of SD are relatively scarce because they are more complex, costly, and have higher safety risks than studies on the ground. One of the biggest difficulties is that the environmental conditions cannot be controlled. This is particularly a problem with investigating visual illusions, such as cloud leans, which depend on weather. Consequently, in-flight studies usually focus on vestibular SD, where the outside visual references are blocked by putting the participant "under the hood." A problem with these studies is to generate the vestibular stimulus in a consistent way, especially when the maneuvers are flown manually. Turbulence may also affect the vestibular stimulus. Furthermore, aircraft motions may not be recorded automatically, so that one needs to install an inertial measurement unit and, for example, a camera to record the participant's response.

Psychophysical Research

Knowledge of the operational range of the sensory systems is fundamental for our understanding of the etiology of SD. Psychophysical experiments can provide insight into stimulus–response relationships in terms of perception threshold, bias (constant error), accuracy (variable error), and the frequency response (gain and phase behavior at different stimulus frequencies). These insights help understand the flight conditions that may lead to SD.

Perception Threshold

According to signal detection theory (Macmillan & Creelman, 2005) a perception threshold can be defined as the stimulus value that is perceived with a significantly higher probability than chance (i.e., pure guessing). Usually, a threshold is determined by fitting a cumulative Gaussian distribution, or psychometric curve, through the proportion of positive responses to a range of stimuli of increasing amplitude. A detection threshold requires a *detection* task ("Do I feel rotation or not?"). Because vestibular stimuli can be bidirectional (left/right, up/down), it may also be interesting to use a *recognition* task ("Do I feel rotation to the left/right?"). Vestibular recognition thresholds are higher than detection thresholds, as shown by Chaudhuri et al. (2013), who found a mean yaw recognition threshold of four participants to be 1.15 deg/s, whereas the mean detection threshold was 0.015 deg/s.

Because of the duration of motion stimuli, or flight profiles, it can take considerably more time to determine a vestibular threshold than, for example, an auditory threshold using brief sound signals. Therefore, vestibular experiments may induce fatigue, inattention, or even motion sickness in participants, and it is recommended to limit the number of stimulus repetitions. This can be done by using a one-interval design instead of a two-interval design (Merfeld, 2011). In the former, participants must report whether or not they perceived a stimulus in each interval, whereas in the latter, they must report in which of two consecutive intervals they perceive self-motion. Another way to reduce the number of repetitions is using adaptive, rather than constant stimuli. Constant stimuli are predetermined by the experimenter, which requires prior knowledge of the response distribution. Without such prior knowledge, the threshold may fall outside the stimulus range. Adaptive methods, such as a *staircase*, do not have this disadvantage because they adapt the stimulus based on the response in the previous trial. This way the stimulus efficiently converges to the threshold value.

As an illustration, Grabherr et al. (2008) used a three-down, one-up staircase paradigm to measure the yaw perception threshold for single cycles of sinusoidal acceleration stimuli with different frequencies (0.05–5 Hz). The perception threshold was highest (2.8 deg/s) at 0.05 Hz, and increased to about 0.6 deg/s at 0.5 Hz. At higher frequencies, the threshold remained constant, in agreement with the high-pass filter characteristics of the semicircular canals.

As a final note on vestibular thresholds, Zaichik et al. (1999) found higher-motion thresholds in the presence of motions in other degrees of freedom (e.g., the threshold for pitch rotation increased with heave motion intensity). This is in accordance with a psychophysical principle, known as Weber-Fechner's law, stating that the "just noticeable difference" (JND), or the smallest difference between two stimuli that can be perceived, increases proportionally with the size of the reference stimulus.

Magnitude Estimation

Because of the time needed for measuring vestibular thresholds, magnitude estimation may be more suitable when investigating a variety of stimuli, or combinations of stimuli (e.g., visual and vestibular). Rather than a minimum stimulus value, magnitude estimation provides a direct measure of the intensity of the perceived motion. Because humans are poor in estimating self-motion in absolute sense (e.g., linear velocity in m/s, or self-tilt in degrees), a labeled rating scale may be useful (with a range of labels such as *none – weak – moderate – strong*). Alternatively, the perceived magnitude of test stimuli can be compared with that of a reference stimulus, which is given an arbitrary value (e.g., Collins, 1968), although care should be taken that participants do not gradually *recalibrate* the reference stimulus during the experiment. Magnitude estimates can be analyzed with a linear model analysis of variance, or a non-parametric method (e.g., Kruskal–Wallis test), depending on whether the responses are obtained by means of an ordinal or categorical scale.

Wickens et al. (2006) measured the somatogyral illusion by asking the participants to continuously indicate the magnitude of their perceived self-rotation in either direction using an analogue slider with a scale of 0–9, where 4.5 indicated *no rotation perceived*. The time history of the slider position reflected the dynamics of the response (indicated by the authors as "time to subjective stationarity"). In addition, participants verbally expressed the magnitude of the turning sensation in the test runs on a subjective scale of 1–10, relative to a "10" rating in the initial condition.

Subjective Vertical (SV)

The perceived body orientation relative to gravity, also referred to as "subjective vertical" (SV), is often measured by aligning a hand-held rod (e.g., Groen et al., 2002) or visual line (e.g., Vingerhoets et al., 2007) parallel to the perceived vertical, or *pointing up*. Alternatively, verbal judgments can be collected in degrees, or using a clock scale, where the body is imagined as the minute hand (e.g., Van Beuzekom & Van Gisbergen 2000). Laboratory studies have shown that SV settings in the dark are accurate in an upright position, but at larger body tilt (> 30 deg) settings systematically deviate in the direction of body tilt (Bischof, 1978). This constant error is known as the "Aubert" or "A-effect," and is explained by considering the SV as a vector sum of a vestibular and visual vector, in combination with an *idiotropic* vector that is defined by the own longitudinal body axis (Groen et al., 2002; Mittelstaedt, 1983).

De Winkel et al. (2012) investigated the SV under reduced gravity levels in parabolic flight. While lying on their side, participants used a trackball finger mouse to align a visual rod inside an HMD with the perceived direction of up. The initial orientation of the visual rod was randomized between trials. Movements of the HMD relative to the head were minimized using a customized bite board. The four different gravity levels (0 g, 0.16 g, 0.38 g, and 1 g) were logged by accelerometers mounted on the floor of the airplane. The data were used to fit psychometric curves, showing that, on average, gravity only affected the SV when it exceeded 0.3 g: At lower gravity levels, the SV was aligned with the longitudinal body axis (i.e., the idiotropic vector).

Self-Nulling

An active way to estimate the perceived motion is by asking participants to cancel or *null* the motion sensation by controlling the motion device. For example, Van Erp et al. (2006) used this approach to measure the somatogyral illusion on a rotating chair. They induced an illusory after-sensation by a sudden stop after a period of constant yaw rotation. Immediately after the stop, the participants were given active control over the yaw motion, and instructed to maintain a constant heading. A random disturbance signal was added to the chair's motion to make sure that participants would engage in the control task. Nooij & Groen (2011) used self-mulling to measure the post-roll illusion in a simulated flight scenario. Immediately after a roll maneuver the pilot was instructed to "maintain constant roll angle" without the help of cockpit instruments. Also in this case a disturbance signal was added to the simulator (roll) motion to mask any vibrations that could reveal whether the cabin was actually moving or not. In addition, white noise was presented through earphones to mask any auditory cues. In 68 % of trials, the participants corrected for the aftersensation by initiating a roll motion in the same direction as the preceding roll, causing an overshoot of roll angle. This post-roll effect was dependent on stimulus rate and duration, consistent with the dynamics of the semicircular canals.

Experimental Procedures

In general, in vestibular experiments the participants should not know which stimulus is presented, so that their response is purely based on their perception. The effect of prior expectation was nicely demonstrated by Wertheim et al. (2001) in a study on a linear track. They showed that participants who watched the device before the experiment correctly reported linear fore–aft motion. By contrast, another group of participants who did not see the device beforehand, reported highly variable sensations, including up and down motion. This underlines the importance to manage the participants' expectations in psychophysical experiments. One way of doing this is to present the stimuli in (pseudo-)random order, so that the participant cannot predict the next stimulus. To account for any order effects, it is good to counterbalance stimuli between participants , for example, using a Latin square design. It is also important to reduce secondary cues that can give away the motion stimulus. Visual cues can be removed by blindfolding the participant; and sound cues by using headphones with (white or pink) noise. Wind cues can be masked by long sleeves and gloves.

Depending on the research question or task, SD experiments can use pilots or non-pilots as participants. Although pilots are less easily available, their results are more representative of the target population. In any case, participants in SD studies should have no vestibular disorders, and abstain from alcohol or drugs that affect vestibular functioning (e.g., sleeping pills, or anti-motion sickness medication). It is important to provide clear instructions prior to the experiment to ensure that all participants consistently use the same response strategy. Sometimes participants may be anxious to make errors, or feel "silly" when their response differs from the stimulus. In those cases, it can be helpful to tell them that they "cannot be wrong," because it is their perception that we are interested in and this may vary between people.

Finally, it should be realized that self-motion stimuli (inertial as well as visual) may induce motion sickness. This must be avoided as much as possible, not only for the well-being of the participants, but also because motion sickness can cause demotivation and lethargy, which negatively impacts the results. There are several measures to minimize the risk of motion sickness, such as: keeping the head against a stable head rest to avoid Coriolis effects; limiting the number of motion stimuli; regularly monitoring the perceived level of discomfort; including rest breaks; and selecting only participants who have no history of motion sickness.

Perception Modeling

The results of psychophysical experiments have been used to develop mathematical models of human self-motion (Bos & Bles, 2002; Bos et al., 2008; McGrath et al., 2002; Newman et al., 2012). These models typically consist of transfer functions that describe the sensory dynamics of the semicircular canals and otolith organs, and their interactions. Perception models may support the investigation of SD as contributing factor in aircraft accidents, by comparing time histories of aircraft motion (from the flight data recorder) with the model-predicted perception of that flight profile (Mumaw et al., 2016). An example of a perception-model analysis of a somatogravic illusion during a go-around maneuver is shown in Figure 5.4. It is important that these perception models are supported by quantitative data from psychophysical experiments, such as performed by Gray et al. (2008) regarding the (mis)perception of runway size. In this study, novice pilots performed a visual approach in a flight simulator, and were then asked to judge whether a set of runway images – with different widths – was smaller or larger than the runway they just landed on. The results showed that the touchdown speed was significantly correlated with perceived runway size. This kind of quantitative relationships between a disorienting stimulus (runway width) and the pilots' response (perceived runway size) can be implemented in perception models.

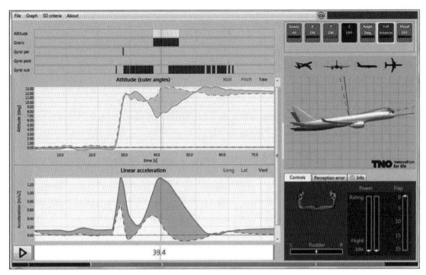

Figure 5.4   Screenshot of the spatial disorientation investigation tool developed by TNO (Mumaw et al., 2016). The time histories on the left show the recorded pitch attitude (solid line in upper plot), and linear acceleration (solid line in bottom plot) of a transport aircraft during a go-around. The dashed lines correspond to the perceived pitch (upper) and linear acceleration (bottom), as computed by the tool's mathematical perception model. The perception error is visualized by the shaded area. At $t = 39.4$ s (vertical line), the perceived pitch attitude is about 6 degrees higher than the actual pitch, a somatogravic illusion. This is also illustrated by the difference between the gray (perceived) and white (actual) aircraft symbol on the right. The bars at the top highlight the automatically detected vestibular illusion, with "gravic" referring to the somatogravic illusion. Reprinted with permission from TNO. © TNO.

Behavioral Responses

Because the main safety risk of SD is that it triggers erroneous control inputs, it is interesting to investigate the impact of SD on pilot control behavior. In a simulator study, Ledegang and Groen (2018) demonstrated that SD effects significantly affected the flight performance of (novice) pilots in a manual flying task. For example, in one phase of the flight the pilots were asked to make a head movement during constant spinning of the simulator. This provoked a vestibular Coriolis illusion, which caused an unintended roll input, and resulted in a substantial deviation in roll angle. Since the Coriolis illusion was noticed by all pilots, this can be considered Type-II SD. In another phase of the flight, the pilots were instructed to look outside for traffic, while they were flying over a sloping cloud deck, presenting a false horizon. This induced an unintended roll input into the direction of the false horizon, even in pilots who were unaware of the SD (Type I).

In the same study, Ledegang and Groen (2018) measured the pilots' instrument scanning by means of gaze tracking. Similar to Cheung and Hofer (2003) they found that the Coriolis illusion caused a delay of the first glance toward the required cockpit instrument. At the same time there was an increased saccadic activity, suggesting that the instrument scan was disturbed by reflexive vestibular eye movements. These results illustrate that gaze behavior can provide relevant information in relation to SD. Apart from measuring a pilot's instrument scan, eye movements can also be used as a more general measure for pilot workload (e.g., De Rivecourt et al., 2008).

Physiological Responses

In many studies, pilots' workload or stress was measured with physiological parameters, such as cardiovascular parameters (heart rate, HR, and heart rate variability, HRV) obtained by electrocardiography (ECG). Today, many biomonitoring devices are available on the customer market, such as sport watches, which monitor heart rate, but it may be unclear how the signal processing is done in these devices. For research purposes it is preferable to record raw signals, and analyze them with known signal-processing algorithms. Other physiological indicators of workload are the galvanic skin response (GSR), the pupil reflex, and respiration frequency. Cheung et al. (2004) found that a false sensation of (simulator) pitch produced systematic changes in mean arterial pressure and HRV, but not in GSR and eye movements. In another study, Westmoreland et al. (2007) found that a Coriolis illusion induced a rise in HR, as well as increased electrodermal response, indicative of enhanced sympathetic activity. Tropper et al. (2009) used physiological measurements to evaluate SD awareness training in a moving base simulator, and found that pilots who received such awareness training had lower HR in a test scenario with unusual attitude recoveries, compared with pilots who did not receive the training (control group).

Some studies examined whether electroencephalography (EEG) can provide markers for SD (Tokumaru et al., 1999; Tropper & Kallus, 2005; Van Orden et al., 2007). In general, EEG signals correlate with overall intracerebral electrical activity. Spectral power analysis of the EEG signal, in particular in the alpha frequency band (8–13 Hz), together with event-related potentials (especially the P300), is seen as an indicator of workload (Brouwer et al., 2012). Van Orden et al. (2007) described that the alpha EEG activity was related to the participants' certainty about their orientation in a

PC-based navigation task. EEG was measured in seated participants who indicated their orientation in a virtual maze at regular intervals. The results showed that alpha EEG activity, measured at the ventral–posterior midline, significantly differed between correct and incorrect responses 500 ms prior to the response. Because only responses were analyzed where the participants were confident about their orientation, even when they were incorrect, the difference in EEG signals resembles Type-I, or unrecognized SD. In another study, EEG alpha band power significantly changed during a vection stimulus (Type-II SD), although response patterns differed between participants (Tokumaru et al. 1999).

Cognitive Performance

There seems to be a two-way interaction between cognitive performance and SD. On the one hand, high cognitive workload can impact the pilot's attention for the flight task and increase their susceptibility for sensory illusions. On the other hand, SD itself can drain cognitive resources according to a principle called "posture first" (Kerr et al., 1985). Gresty et al. (2008) found that a Coriolis sensation (provoked by head movements during constant rotation with 90 deg/s on a rotating chair) negatively affected the performance on a Manikin test, which involves spatial transformation of mental images. The scores were lowest during the initial Coriolis experience, and improved during subsequent exposures, indicating that participants learned to quarantine the disorientating sensation. However, such learning effect may have little meaning for pilots in-flight, when experiencing a single, unexpected SD event.

Webb et al. (2012) investigated the cognitive performance of 36 military helicopter pilots who were actively engaged in oriented and disorientation scenarios in a flight simulator. Cognitive performance was measured with two secondary tests for working memory, the digit span test and a number addition test. The tests were presented aurally (hands free), so that they did not interfere with the control of the aircraft. In the SD scenario, the occurrence of roll reversal errors confirmed that pilots were disoriented. Performance on both cognitive tests (mean reaction time and accuracy) was significantly worse in this SD scenario compared with the orientation scenarios.

Situational awareness (SA) is a particularly interesting construct in relation to SD. According to the model of Endsley (1999), three levels of SA can be distinguished: perception (Level 1), comprehension and meaning (Level 2), and projection of the near future (Level 3). One way to measure SA is the Situation Awareness Global Assessment Technique (SAGAT; Endsley, 2000). The method requires the participant to fill in a query at regular intervals, for which the simulation must be frozen. When the scenario does not allow for these interruptions, the post-trial *situation awareness rating technique* (SART) may also be considered (Taylor, 2011). This method collects subjective self-ratings on 10 different dimensions on a 7-point rating scale (1=*low*, 7=*high*) about the performance of the preceding task, such as attention, perceived complexity of the situation, and arousal, etc.

Emotional Responses

Loss of control in flight (LOC-I) accidents often involve a *startle factor* in response to an unexpected event. Surprising situations can make it difficult for the flight crew to find the right recovery strategy (Landman et al., 2017a). This was demonstrated in two different simulator studies where airline pilots had difficulties in applying the correct recovery procedure in an unexpected aerodynamic stall, which they had practiced in a simulator session just before the test (Landman et al., 2017b; Schroeder et al., 2014). SD can be a contributory factor to LOC-I accidents where it adds to the flight crew's confusion (Mumaw et al., 2016).

It can be difficult to measure the effects of an emotional response on the pilot's flight performance, because as long as certain parameters stay within safe margins it may be considered good performance. Therefore, Landman et al. (2017b) used the number of slips in the recovery procedure, and found that surprise resulted in significantly worse adherence to the procedure (e.g., [1] "disengage autothrottle", [2] "start with pitch-down control"). Subjectively, startle or surprise can be measured on a labeled rating scale or Likert scale. In one study, Landman et al. (2018) used a 5-point labeled rating scale (1=*not at all*, 5=*extremely*) to answer questions such as: "How surprised were you when you discovered the issue?" Landman et al. (2017b) used an 11-point Likert-type scale to collect the level of perceived anxiety, surprise, startle, and confusion. The unexpected stall event resulted in a 7-fold higher surprise rating compared with the anticipated condition. In the surprise condition the electrodermal response (GSR) was also significantly greater than in the anticipation condition. Both outcomes served as manipulation check, confirming that pilots were effectively surprised by the unexpected stall event.

Countermeasures

An important area of research concerns the validation of potential counter-measures against SD, such as special display symbology to support helicopter pilots during brownout landings (Szoboszlay et al., 2009), or peripheral displays to provide a more intuitive sense of motion to the pilot (Eriksson & Van Hofsten, 2002; Malcolm, 1984). In addition to visual countermeasures, tactile feedback may also be effective in increasing a pilot's awareness of the aircraft's motion or orientation (e.g., Brill et al., 2014; Rupert, 2000). In a laboratory study with a rotating chair, Cheung and Hofer (2007) showed that a tactile garment did not produce sensations of vection, but it did provide a clear sense of direction. This sense of direction was exploited by Bos et al. (2005), showing that participants could maintain a stable orientation (self-nulling task) with the help of a tactile direction cue around their waist, despite strong after-sensations of turning after a sudden stop of the rotation chair. Jansen et al. (2008) showed the usefulness of a tactile flight suit as a pilot support tool for landing in degraded visual environments (Figure 5.5). The tactile suit had a vertical array of vibrating elements (*tactors*), to indicate (relative) height above terrain, and a horizontal array to indicate ground speed (in particular lateral drift). The test flight showed that, whereas landings without external references and only instruments were unacceptable, the pilot was able to make landings when he or she was guided by tactile feedback on vertical and lateral motion.

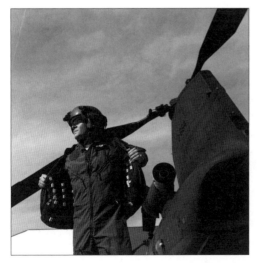

Figure 5.5   Tactile flight suit for helicopter pilots. Reprinted with permission from TNO. © TNO.

Conclusion

This chapter only scratched the surface of applicable research methods. It is recommended to consult specific literature or textbooks to find more details about a useful method related to the research question at hand. Future SD research could address the consequences of increasing levels of automation in next-generation cockpits, as well as the use of new technologies, such as virtual reality (VR) or augmented reality (AR). It is important to understand how these developments will affect a pilot's situational awareness, information processing, man–machine teaming, and transition of control. In conclusion, SD is a multidisciplinary research field that improves aviation safety, by developing knowledge, training programs, and countermeasures, which should ultimately help pilots to recognize and avoid SD.

References

Asch, S. E., & Witkin, H. A. (1948). Studies in space orientation. I. Perception of the upright with displaced visual fields. *Journal of Experimental Psychology, 38*(3), 325–337. https://doi.org/10.1037/h0057855

Allison, R. S., Howard, I. P., & Zacher, J. E. (1999). Effect of field size, head motion, and rotational velocity on roll vection and illusory self-tilt in a tumbling room. *Perception, 28*(3), 299–306. https://doi.org/10.1068/p2891

Beringer, D. B., Williges, R. C., & Roscoe, S. N. (1975). The transition of experienced pilots to a frequency-separated aircraft attitude display. *Human Factors, 17*(4), 401–414. https://doi.org/10.1177/001872087501700411

Bischof, N. (1978). Optic-vestibular orientation to the vertical. In H. H. Kornhuber (Ed.), *Handbook of sensory physiology VI/2: Vestibular system* (pp. 155–190). Springer. https://doi.org/10.1007/978-3-642-65920-1_2

Bles, W., & Groen, E. (2009). The DESDEMONA motion facility: Applications for space research. *Microgravity Science and Technology, 21*(4), 281–286. https://doi.org/10.1007/s12217-009-9120-1

Bos, J. E., & Bles, W. (2002). Theoretical considerations on canal-otolith interaction and an observer model. *Biological Cybernetics, 86*(3), 191–207. https://doi.org/10.1007/s00422-001-0289-7

Bos, J. E., Bles, W., & Groen, E. L. (2008). A theory on visually induced motion sickness. *Displays, 29*(2), 47–57. https://doi.org/10.1016/j.displa.2007.09.002

Bos, J. E., Van Erp, J., Groen, E. L., & Van Veen, H. J. A. C. (2005). Vestibulo-tactile interactions regarding motion perception and eye movements in yaw. *Journal of Vestibular Research: Equilibrium and Orientation, 15*(3), 149–160.

Brill, J. C., Lawson, B. D., & Rupert, A. H. (2014). Tactile situation awareness system (TSAS) as a compensatory aid for sensory loss. *Proceedings of the Human Factors and Ergonomics Society Annual Meeting, 58*(1), 1028–1032. https://doi.org/10.1177/1541931214581215

Brouwer, A. M., Hogervorst, M. A., & Van Erp, J. B. F. (2012). Estimating workload using EEG spectral power and ERPs in the n-back task. *Journal of Neural Engineering, 9*(4), 1-14. https://doi.org/10.1088/1741-2560/9/4/045008

Chaudhuri, S. E., Karmali, F., & Merfeld, D. M. (2013). Whole body motion-detection tasks can yield much lower thresholds than direction-recognition tasks: Implications for the role of vibration. *Journal of Neurophysiology, 110*(12), 2764-2772. https://doi.org/10.1152/jn.00091.2013

Cheung, B., & Hofer, K. (2003). Eye tracking, point of gaze, and performance degradation during disorientation. *Aviation, Space, and Environmental Medicine, 74*(1), 11-20.

Cheung, B., & Hofer, K. (2007). Tactile cueing vs. vestibular sensation and nystagmus during yaw rotation. *Aviation, Space, and Environmental Medicine, 78*(8), 756-63.

Cheung, B., Hofer, K., Heskin, R., & Smith, A. (2004). Physiological and behavioral responses to an exposure of pitch illusion in the simulator. *Aviation, Space, and Environmental Medicine, 75*(8), 657-665.

Cohen, M. M. (1976). Disorienting effects of aircraft catapult launchings II. Visual and postural contributions. *Aviation, Space, and Environmental Medicine, 47*(1), 39-41.

Cohen, M. M., Crosbie, R. J., & Blackburn, L. H. (1973). Disorienting effects of aircraft catapult launchings. *Aviation, Space, and Environmental Medicine, 44*(1), 37-39.

Collins, W. E. (1968). Coriolis vestibular stimulation and the influence of different visual surrounds. *Aerospace Medicine, 39*(2), 125-130.

Correia Grácio, B. J., De Winkel, K. N., Groen, E. L., Wentink, M., & Bos, J. E. (2013). The time constant of the somatogravic illusion. *Experimental Brain Research, 224*(3), 313-321. https://doi.org/10.1007/s00221-012-3313-3

De Rivecourt, M., Kuperus, M. N., Post, W. J., & Mulder, L. J. M. (2008). Cardiovascular and eye activity measures as indices for momentary changes in mental effort during simulated flight. *Ergonomics, 51*(9), 1295-1319. https://doi.org/10.1080/00140130802120267

De Winkel, K. N., Clément, G., Groen, E. L., & Werkhoven, P. J. (2012). The perception of verticality in lunar and Martian gravity conditions. *Neuroscience Letters, 529*(1), 7-11. https://doi.org/10.1016/j.neulet.2012.09.026

Dichgans, J., & Brandt, T. (1978). Visual-vestibular interaction: Effects on self-motion, perception and postural control. In R. Held, H. W. Leibowitz, & H.-L. Teuber (Eds.), *Handbook of sensory physiology, Vol. 8: Perception* (pp. 755-804). Springer. https://doi.org/10.1007/978-3-642-46354-9_25

Endsley, M. R. (1999). Situation awareness in aviation systems. In D. J. Garland, J. A. Wise, & V. D. Hopkin (Eds.), *Human factors in transportation. Handbook of aviation human factors* (pp. 257-276). Lawrence Erlbaum Associates Publishers.

Endsley, M. R. (2000). Direct measurement of situation awareness: Validity and use of SAGAT. In M. R. Endsley & D. J. Garland (Eds.), *Situation awareness analysis and measurement* (pp. 147-174). Lawrence Erlbaum Associates. https://www.researchgate.net/publication/245934995_Direct_Measurement_of_Situation_Awareness_Validity_and_Use_of_SAGAT

Eriksson, L., & Von Hofsten, C. (2002, April). *On the possibility of counteracting or reducing G-induced spatial disorientation with visual displays.* Paper presented at the Spatial Disorientation in Military Vehicles: Causes, Consequences and Cures. NATO-RTO Human Factors & Medicine Panel Symposium, La Coruna, Spain.

Ercoline, W. R., Devilbiss, C. A., Yauch, D. W., & Brown, D. L. (2000). Post-roll effects on attitude perception: "The Gillingham Illusion." *Aviation, Space, and Environmental Medicine, 71*(5), 489–495.

Grabherr, L., Nicoucar, K., Mast, F. W., & Merfeld, D. M. (2008). Vestibular thresholds for yaw rotation about an earth-vertical axis as a function of frequency. *Experimental Brain Research, 186*(4), 677–681. https://doi.org/10.1007/s00221-008-1350-8

Gray, R., Navia, J. A., & Allsop, J. (2008). Action-specific effects in aviation: What determines judged runway size? *Perception, 43*, 145–154. https://doi.org/10.1068/p7601

Gresty, M. A., Golding, J. F., Le, H., & Nightingale, K. (2008). Cognitive impairment by spatial disorientation. *Aviation, Space, and Environmental Medicine, 79*(2), 105–111. https://doi.org/10.3357/asem.2143.2008

Groen, E. L., & Bles, W. (2004). How to use body tilt for the simulation of linear self-motion. *Journal of Vestibular Research, 14*(5), 375–385.

Groen, E. L., Jenkin, H. L., & Howard, I. P. (2002). Perception of self-tilt in a true and illusory vertical plane. *Perception, 31*(12), 1477–1490. https://doi.org/10.1068/p3330

Groen, E. L., Smaili, M. H., & Hosman, R. J. A. W. (2007). Perception model analysis of flight simulator motion for a decrab maneuver. *Journal of Aircraft, 44*(2), 427–435. https://doi.org/10.2514/1.22872

Groen, E. L., Valenti Clari, M. S. V., & Hosman, R. J. A. W. (2001). Evaluation of perceived motion during a simulated takeoff run. *Journal of Aircraft, 38*(4), 600–606. https://doi.org/10.2514/2.2827

Guedry, F. E. (1974). Psychophysics of vestibular sensation. In H. H. Kornhuber (Eds.), *Vestibular system part 2: Psychophysics, applied aspects and general interpretations. Handbook of sensory physiology, Vol. 6/2*. Springer. https://doi.org/10.1007/978-3-642-65920-1_1

Guedry, F. E., Jr., & Benson, A. J. (1978). Coriolis cross-coupling effects: Disorienting and nauseogenic or not? *Aviation, Space, and Environmental Medicine, 49*(1), 29–35.

Howard, I. P., & Childerson, L. (1994). The contribution of motion, the visual frame, and visual polarity to sensations of body tilt. *Perception, 23*(7), 753–762. https://doi.org/10.1068/p230753

Jansen, C., Wennemers, A., Vos, W., & Groen, E. (2008). FlyTact: A tactile display improves a helicopter pilot's landing performance in degraded visual environments. In M. Ferre (Ed.), *Haptics: Perception, devices and scenarios. EuroHaptics 2008. Lecture Notes in Computer Science: Vol. 5024* (pp. 867–875). https://doi.org/10.1007/978-3-540-69057-3_109

Kallus, W., Tropper, K., & Boucsein, W. (2011). The importance of motion cues in spatial disorientation training for VFR-Pilots. *International Journal of Aviation Psychology, 21*(2), 135–152. https://doi.org/10.1080/10508414.2011.556458

Kerr, B., Condon, S. M., & McDonald, L. A. (1985). Cognitive spatial processing and the regulation of posture. *Journal of Experimental Psychology: Human Perception and Performance, 11*(5), 617–622. https://doi.org/10.1037//0096-1523.11.5.617

Klyde, D. H., Lampton, A. K., & Schulze, P. C. (2016, January). *Development of spatial disorientation demonstration scenarios for commercial pilot training. AIAA 2016-1180*. Paper presentation. AIAA Modeling and Simulation Technologies Conference, San Diego, CA. https://doi.org/10.2514/6.2016-1180

Landman, A., Davies, S., Groen, E. L., Van Paassen, M. M., Lawson, N. J., Bronkhorst, A. W., & Mulder, M. (2019). In-flight spatial disorientation induces roll reversal errors when using the attitude indicator. *Applied Ergonomics, 81*, 102905. https://doi.org/10.1016/j.apergo.2019.102905

Landman, A., Groen, E. L., Van Paassen, M. M., Bronkhorst, A. W., & Mulder, M. (2017a). Dealing with unexpected events on the flight deck: A conceptual model of startle and surprise. *Human factors, 59*(8), 1161-1172. https://doi.org/10.1177/0018720817723428

Landman, A., Groen, E. L., Van Paassen, M. M., Bronkhorst, A. W., & Mulder, M. (2017b). The influence of surprise on upset recovery performance in airline pilots. *International Journal of Aerospace Psychology, 27*(1-2), 2-14. https://doi.org/10.1080/10508414.2017.1365610

Landman, A., Oorschot, P., Van Paassen, M. M., Groen, E. L., Bronkhorst, A. W., & Mulder, M. (2018). Training pilots for unexpected events: A simulator study on the advantage of unpredictable and variable scenarios. *Human Factors, 60*(6), 793-805. https://doi.org/10.1177/0018720818779928

Ledegang, W. D., & Groen, E. L. (2015). Stall recovery in a centrifuge-based flight simulator with an extended aerodynamic model. *The International Journal of Aviation Psychology, 25*(2), 122-140. https://doi.org/10.1080/10508414.2015.1131085

Ledegang, W. D., & Groen, E. L. (2018). Spatial disorientation influences on pilots' visual scanning and flight performance. *Aerospace Medicine and Human Performance, 89*(10), 873-882. https://doi.org/10.3357/AMHP.5109.2018

Macmillan, N. A., & Creelman, C. D. (2005). *Detection theory: A user's guide* (2nd ed.). Psychological Press. https://doi.org/10.4324/9781410611147

Malcik, V. (1968). Performance decrement in a flight simulator due to galvanic stimulation of the vestibular organ and its validity for success in flight training. *Aerospace Medicine, 39*(9), 941-943.

Malcolm, R. (1984). Pilot disorientation and the use of a peripheral vision display. *Aviation, Space, and Environmental Medicine, 55*, 231-238.

McCarthy, G. W., & Stott, J. R. R. (1994). In flight verification of the inversion illusion. *Aviation, Space, and Environmental Medicine, 65*(4), 341-344.

McGrath, B., Rupert, A. H., & Guedry, F. E. (2002, April). *Analysis of spatial disorientation mishaps in the US Navy*. Paper presented at the Spatial Disorientation in Military Vehicles: Causes, Consequences and Cures, NATO-RTO Human Factors & Medicine Panel Symposium, La Coruna, Spain.

Melcher, G. A. & Henn, V. (1981). The latency of circular vection during different accelerations of the optokinetic stimulus. *Perception and Psychophysics, 30*(6), 552-556. https://doi.org/10.3758/BF03202009

Merfeld, D. M. (2011). Signal detection theory and vestibular thresholds: I. Basic theory and practical considerations. *Experimental Brain Research, 210*, 389-405. https://doi.org/10.1007/s00221-011-2557-7

Mittelstaedt, H. (1983). A new solution to the subjective vertical. *Naturwissenschaften, 70*, 272-281. https://doi.org/10.1007/BF00404833

Moore, S. T., Dilda, V., & MacDougall, H. G. (2011). Galvanic vestibular stimulation as an analogue of spatial disorientation after spaceflight. *Aviation, Space, and Environmental Medicine, 82*(5), 535-542. https://doi.org/10.3357/ASEM.2942.2011

Müller, S., Roche, F., & Manzey, D. (2019). Attitude indicator format: How difficult is the transition between different reference systems? *Aviation Psychology and Applied Human Factors, 9*(2), 95-105. https://doi.org/10.1027/2192-0923/a000168

Mumaw, R. J., Groen, E., Fucke, L., Anderson, R., Bos, J., & Houben, M. (2016). A new tool for analyzing the potential influence of vestibular illusions. *ISASI Forum, January–March,* 6–12.

Newman, M. C., Lawson, B. D., Rupert, A. H., & McGrath, B. J. (2012, August). *The role of perceptual modeling in the understanding of spatial disorientation during flight and ground-based simulator training.* Paper presented at the AIAA Modeling and Simulation Technologies Conference, Minneapolis, MN. https://doi.org/10.2514/6.2012-5009

Nooij, S. A. E., & Groen, E. L. (2011). Rolling into spatial disorientation: simulator demonstration of the post-roll (Gillingham) illusion. *Aviation, Space, and Environmental Medicine, 82*(5), 505–512. https://doi.org/10.3357/ASEM.2946.2011

Previc, F. H., & Ercoline, W. R. (2004). *Spatial disorientation in aviation.* American Institute of Astronautics and Aeronautics. https://doi.org/10.2514/4.866708

Previc, F. H., Ercoline, W. R., Evans, R. H., Dillon, N., & Lopez, N., (2007). Simulator induced spatial disorientation: Effects of age, sleep deprivation, and type of conflict. *Aviation, Space, and Environmental Medicine, 78*(5), 470–477.

Previc, F. H., Lopez, N., Ercoline, W. R., Daluz, C. M., & Workman, A. J. (2009). The effects of sleep deprivation on flight performance, instrument scanning, and physiological arousal in pilots. *International Journal of Aviation Psychology, 19*(4), 326–346. https://doi.org/10.1080/10508410903187562

Previc, F. H., Varner, D., & Gillingham, K. (1992). Visual scene effects on the somatogravic illusion. *Aviation, Space, and Environmental Medicine, 63,* 1060–1064.

Rupert, A. H. (2000). An instrument solution for reducing spatial disorientation mishaps: A more 'natural approach to maintaining spatial orientation. *IEEE Engineering in Medicine and Biology Magazine, 19*(2), 71–80. https://doi.org/10.1109/51.827409

Schroeder, J. A., Bürki-Cohen, J., Shikany, D. A., Gingras, D. R., Desrochers, P. (2014, January). *An evaluation of several stall models for commercial transport training.* Paper presented at the AIAA Modeling and Simulation Technologies Conference, Washington, DC. https://doi.org/10.2514/6.2014-1002

Stott, J. R. R. (2013). Orientation and disorientation in aviation. *Extreme Physiology & Medicine, 2*(2), 1–11. https://doi.org/10.1186/2046-7648-2-2

Szoboszlay, Z. P., Turpin, T. S., & Mckinley, R. A. (2009, May). *Symbology for brown-out landings: The first simulation for the 3D-LZ program.* Paper presented at the American Helicopter Society 65th Annual Forum, Grapevine, TX.

Taylor, R. M. (2011). Situational Awareness Rating Technique (Sart): The development of a tool for aircrew systems design. In E. Salas & A. S. Dietz (Eds.), *Situational awareness* (pp. 111–128). Routledge. https://doi.org/10.4324/9781315087924

Tokumaru, O., Kaida, K., Ashida, H., Mizumoto, C., & Tatsuno, J. (1998). Visual influence on the magnitude of somatogravic illusion evoked in advanced spatial disorientation demonstrator. *Aviation, Space, and Environmental Medicine, 69*(2), 111–116.

Tokumaru, O., Kaida, K., Ashida, H., Yoneda, I., & Tatsuno, J. (1999). EEG topographical analysis of spatial disorientation. *Aviation, Space, and Environmental Medicine, 70*(3), 256–263.

Tropper, K. & Kallus, K. W. (2005, April). *Disorientation in VFR Pilots: Flight performance and psychophysiological changes during a flight simulator training.* Paper presented at the 13th International Symposium on Aviation Psychology, Oklahoma City, OK.

Tropper, K., Kallus, W., & Boucsein, W. (2009). Psychophysiological evaluation of an anti-disorientation training for visual flight rules pilots in a moving base simulator.

International Journal of Aviation Psychology, 19(3), 270–286. https://doi.org/10.1080/10508410902983912

Van Beuzekom, A. D., & Van Gisbergen, J. A. M. (2000). Properties of the internal representation of gravity inferred from spatial-direction and body-tilt estimates. *Journal of Neurophysiology, 84*(1), 11–27. https://doi.org/10.1152/jn.2000.84.1.11

Van Erp, J. B. F., Groen, E. L., Bos, J. E., & Van Veen, H. A. H. C. (2006). A tactile cockpit instrument supports the control of self-motion during spatial disorientation. *Human Factors, 48*(2), 219–228. https://doi.org/10.1518/001872006777724435

Van Orden, K. F., Viirre, E., & Kobus, D. A. (2007). Augmenting task-centered design with operator state assessment technologies. In D. D. Schmorrow, & L. M. Reeves (Eds.), *Foundations of augmented cognition. FAC 2007. Lecture Notes in Computer Science, Vol. 4565* (pp. 212–219), Springer. https://doi.org/10.1007/978-3-540-73216-7_24

Vingerhoets, R. A. A., Van Gisbergen, J. A. M., & Medendorp, W. P. (2007). Verticality perception during off-vertical axis rotation. *Journal of Neurophysiology, 97*, 3256–3268. https://doi.org/10.1152/jn.01333.2006

Webb, C. M., Estrada, A., III, & Kelley, A. M. (2012). The effects of spatial disorientation on cognitive processing. *International Journal of Aviation Psychology, 22*(3), 224–241. https://doi.org/10.1080/10508414.2012.689211

Wertheim, A. H., Mesland, B. S., & Bles, W. (2001). Cognitive suppression of tilt sensations during linear horizontal self-motion in the dark. *Perception, 30*(6), 733–741. https://doi.org/10.1068/p3092

Westmoreland, D., Krell, R. W., & Self, B. P. (2007). Physiological responses to the Coriolis illusion: Effects of head position and vision. *Aviation, Space, and Environmental Medicine, 78*(10), 985–989. https://doi.org/10.3357/asem.2010.2007

Wickens, C. D., Self, B. P., Small, R. L., Williams, C. B., Burrows, C. L., Levinthal, B. R., & Keller, J. W. (2006). Rotation rate and duration effects on the somatogyral illusion. *Aviation, Space, and Environmental Medicine, 77*(12), 1244–1251.

Zaichik, L. E., Rodchenko, V., Rufov, I., Yashin, Y., & White, A. D. (1999, August). *Acceleration perception.* Paper presented at the AIAA Modeling and Simulation Technologies Conference and Exhibit, Portland, OR. https://doi.org/10.2514/6.1999-4334

Chapter 6
Reactivity – The Process Behind the States and Traits

Thomas Uhlig and Christiane Uhlig

Abstract

In the field of applied psychology, the prediction of how a person reacts in a specified setting is of general interest for both practitioners and scientists alike. In aviation and work psychology the prediction of reactions is highlighted in particular in the context of safety management (e.g., risk reduction in high- reliability environments, error management in general). Attempts are made to describe human performance under different conditions and to evaluate psychological concepts that are responsible for it. It is very common to use aspects of personality (traits) or emotion (states) or other concepts for the prediction of performance. Thereby it is assumed that a relatively well-defined psychological "*baseline*" is able not only to predict reactions but also provides evidence for the improvement of performance. There is no doubt about the significant correlations between psychological traits and states and aspects of performance, but in many cases these correlations are not substantial. When looking for solutions that may be suitable to increase the impact of psychological thinking in the context of safety at work, the concept of reactivity is a suitable option. Thereby performance is considered a process that is modulated and mediated by classical as well as newer concepts. The focus of interest lies on the question of how a performance takes place and, what its determinants and influencing factors are, not only on why it takes place. In this chapter reactivity is defined as a biopsychological concept and methodological as well as practical considerations are made.

Keywords: stress, performance, reactivity, emotional state, process analysis

Introduction

In chemistry, reactivity describes the tendency of a molecule or an element to come into contact and react with other molecules and elements. This happens because most of the molecules and elements are eager to achieve a higher level of stability. During the process of reaction, the original structure of the molecules and elements changes and new elements or molecules develop. In medicine, aspects of reactivity are frequently used in the processes of diagnosis and therapy of illness. For example, humans commonly react with increasing levels of inflammatory proteins in the blood plasma after coming into contact with bacteria, viruses, and other microbial agents. In this case, the occurrence of illness is documented regularly by higher levels of the so-called C–reactive protein. If, in addition, other substances also react (i.e., procalcitonin) one is able to define the body's reaction as a consequence of bacterial infection but not a viral or fungal one.

In psychology, however, aspects of reactivity are certainly well-known but somewhat ignored in particular in fields of applied psychology. This may be due to the fact that reactivity in psychology is frequently defined as a synonym of the Hawthorne effect. This definition recognizes in particular a person's reaction in an experimental or laboratory setting. If a person feels they are being watched by others, several psychological processes are initiated as a consequence of that feeling. The Hawthorne effect is a basic paradigm in experimental psychology that has been discussed intensively by Franke and Kaul (1978). Dealing with the Hawthorne effect regularly leads to the acceptance of increasing variances in the data obtained. Since the increasing variances are considered to be present in the experimental as well in the control groups, the Hawthorne effect is seen as a source of increasing noise in the data but not as an effect that has to be operationalized in a differentiated manner.

On the other hand, there is evidence from pharmacology, in particular psychopharmacology, that the feeling of being part of a study or taking a therapeutic drug per se is able to initiate mental processes like changes in well-being or pain. These results originate from the growing research on placebo or nocebo effects (Baethge, 2013). Mental processes are able to induce effects that are similar to a therapy with drugs. These effects can be either positive (placebo) or negative (nocebo). Obviously, it is the feeling of being treated that leads to these effects. This is similar to the feeling of being watched in an experimental situation.

Taken together, all these aspects contribute to the knowledge, that reactivity in psychology is a valuable (research) tool, and not simply a nice toy.

Definition of Reactivity

More than 20 years ago Janke and Kallus (1995) published a remarkable and elaborate article dedicated to aspects of reactivity in a German encyclopedia of psychology. This article was frequently cited in handbooks of statistics and methods of measurement in psychology. A similar article dedicated to aspects of stress and anxiety in anesthesiology was published some years later (Kallus, 1997). Dealing with reactivity is part of daily psychological work both in research and in the applied field.

In general, reactivity should be seen as a tendency of an individual to react on external and/or internal stimuli. This tendency is either shorter lasting, or specific for an actual state or situation. It may be longer lasting and thus represent stable reactions over time and situations.

The purpose of all efforts in the context of reactivity is the intention of the individual to regain a stable and homeostatic state that has been lost due to the stimulus effects. The efforts either restore the former baseline or lead to an alternative state that is considered to be more suitable for the adaption to the stimulus effects. In this context, adaption means a decreasing reaction of an individual due to a continuous presentation of a stimulus during a period of time. Alternatively, habituation means a decreasing reaction of an individual due to several presentations of the same stimulus over time (Janke, 1974). These basic principles of reactivity should be accepted in any case when questions of different actions in different individuals arise.

Reactivity includes aspects of mood, cognition, and behavior as well as humoral, immunological, or muscular aspects. Regulatory processes of the central and peripheral nervous system are also included. From a biopsychological point of view, reactivity summarizes at least the following aspects of individual reactions (Janke & Kallus, 1995): responsiveness and deflection capability of an organism, adaptability, robustness, and a tendency to change conditions actively when a (stressful) stimulus occurs.

Just by mentioning these few considerations on reactivity it becomes clear that the construct is complex and somewhat puzzling. Therefore, it is necessary to introduce a pragmatic approach that allows psychologists in the applied field to deal with the construct. This approach should be not too sophisticated but should also be suitable to accept and integrate influences of reactivity in daily work.

Reactivity in Applied Psychology

In the field of applied psychology, the prediction of how a person reacts in a specified setting is of general interest for practitioners and for scientists alike. In aviation and work psychology the prediction of reactions is highlighted in particular in the context of safety management (e.g., risk reduction in high/reliability environments, error management in general). Attempts are made to describe human performance under different conditions and to evaluate psychological concepts that are responsible for it. It is very common to use aspects of personality (traits) or emotion (states) or other concepts for the prediction of performance. Thereby it is assumed that a relatively well-defined psychological baseline is able not only to predict reactions but also provides evidence for the improvement of performance.

There is no doubt about the correlations between psychological traits and states and aspects of performance, but in many cases these correlations are not substantial. For example, a significant correlation of 0.3 between neuroticism and performance under stress means a common variance of these factors of less than 10 %. This is far below the standards used in other fields of work psychology, technical disciplines, or engineering.

When looking for solutions that may be suitable to increase the impact of psychological thinking in the context of safety at work, the concept of reactivity can be an option. Thereby, performance is considered as a process that is modulated and mediated by reactivity, as defined earlier. The focus of interest lies in the question of how performance takes place and what its determinants and influencing factors are.

Aspects of Sensitivity and Specificity of Indicators

In almost every context, psychologists look for indicators of experience and behavior that are able to depict psychological states and processes. These indicators should be easy to define and easy to obtain and should at least have a valuable validity to explain the constructs of interest. A practitioner in aviation psychology, for example, should explore the scientific psychological portfolio to find out which of the numerous and established indicators may be helpful for the explanation of processes in practice. This leads to the concepts of sensitivity and specificity of an indicator by which almost every indicator can be classified as suitable or not for the explanation of an individual reaction in a defined setting. Thus one should be aware not only of the indicators themselves but also of their kinetics during a process.

In general, sensitivity means the ability of an indicator to represent changes in an individual's reaction almost simultaneously. For example, an individual's increasing heart rate is an accepted indicator of increasing activation. In addition, specificity means the ability of an indicator to depict a state or process as precisely as possible. For example, an individual's increasing heart rate is not suitable for the explanation of chronic stress, whereas hormones of the hypothalamic–pituitary–adrenergic axis are, in particular the so-called cortisol awakening response (Chida & Steptoe, 2008).

In psychology the specificity of an indicator should also be discussed with regard to superordinate concepts such as individual specificity, situational specificity, and stimulus specificity. Individual specificity determines a person's specific tendencies of reactivity independent of situation or type of stimulus. For example, Person A always has a headache in almost every stressful situation, whereas Person B always experiences nausea or vomiting. Situational specificity describes tendencies of reaction as characteristic of a well-defined situation. For example, small talk with an academic has almost no influence on a student's activation whereas the same talk on the same topics leads to an extreme increase in activation if it takes place during an examination. Finally, specificity of a stimulus means that a stimulus is able to increase reactivity independent of a person's tendencies to react and independent of situational aspects. For instance, white noise can be used as a stressor for almost every person in almost every situation. By using mathematical procedures, the sensitivity and specificity of an indicator can be calculated with regard to the psychological construct that has been investigated.

Hinz et al. (2002) measured physiological and psychological variables of students in comparable stress conditions such as mental arithmetic tasks, blood-taking, free speech, cold-pressor test. For physiological variables, Hinz and colleagues (2002) found that 23–29 % of variance was specific to the individual, 5–19 % was specific to the stimulus, and 21 % was specific to the motivation. Overall, 6–11 % of the variance of psychological variables was attributed to the individual, 1–11 % was stimulus-specific, and 10 % was motivation-specific (Hinz et al., 2002). These results were reliable over a period of several weeks. In addition, Hinz et al. (2002) found a stable individual-specific response pattern in physiological variables in one fourth of the participants.

The classic way to determine whether an indicator has an acceptable sensitivity and specificity follows its diagnostic strength. An indicator should be able to divide groups of persons with regard to the availability of a diagnosis (true or false) and, in addition, it should not be prone to errors. This means that a positive prediction of an indicator is indeed positive (true positive) and not negative (false positive). And vice versa this also applies to the prediction as true negative and false negative. The mathematical procedures using data from Figure 6.1 are:

- Sensitivity = $A/(A+C) \times 100$
- Specificity = $D/(D+B) \times 100$

Since aspects of sensitivity and specificity of an indicator are dependent on one another and it is obviously unrealistic to look for indicators that show both maximal sensitivity and maximal specificity, a compromise is warranted. This compromise lies in the construction of the so-called receiver operating characteristic (ROC) curves (Figure 6.2), which are used to quan-

	Truth		
	Right	False	
Test Result	A	B	Test positive
	C	D	Test negative
	Truth Valid	Truth Non-valid	Total

Figure 6.1   The calculation of sensitivity and specificity.

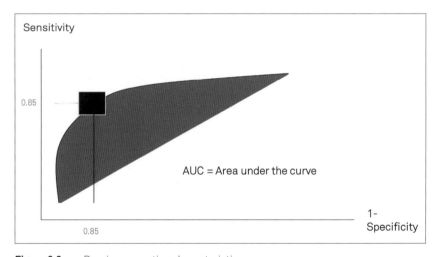

Figure 6.2   Receiver operating characteristic curves.

tify the diagnostic power an indicator has based on its sensitivity and specificity.

The use of ROC curves makes it possible to compare a number of indicators with one another as well as the range of values of an indicator, which may be suitable to distinguish whether a diagnosis made should be taken or not. The selection of suitable indicators with acceptable and valuable sensitivity and specificity is the basis of a structured analysis of reactivity aspects.

Foerster et al. (1983a, 1983b) highlighted the importance of specificity of psychophysiological responses to behavioral stimuli for basic and applied psychophysiological research. Research shows that on single parameters, level scores have a higher profile reliability than change scores (Hinz et al.,

2002). In addition, the stability of situational response patterns is high for data aggregated across subjects and low for individual response patterns (Hinz et al., 2002). Inconsistencies of variance estimates and the relationship between temporal stability, consistency, and covariation of physiological variables need to be addressed (Hinz et al., 2002).

Burt and Obradovic (2013) recommended an increased attention to the ubiquitous nature of measurement error in observed variables and the importance of employing latent variable models when possible. Furthermore, the specification of theories relating to the construct of reactivity, especially in regard to the distinction between baseline arousal, and to change over time in broader systems of variables is recommended. These recommendations lead to discussions on aspects of the law of initial values.

The Law of Initial Values

Discussions on the law of initial values have a long history in psychology research and practice. Starting with the definition by Wilder (1931), several authors (Janke, 1974; Kallus 1992, 1997) addressed the associated methodological and statistical issues.

To date, there is no doubt that the correlation between change and initial levels of an indicator is important to avoid systematic errors in decision-making based on psychological evidence. The influence of initial values on change has to be proven individually in any case. A change in variance between pre- and posttest levels or a regression of measurements to the mean can be used as a preliminary hint that a reaction is systematically influenced by the initial value (Jamieson, 1993). More generally the correlation between change and initial levels is affected by measurement errors (that shows the importance of sensitivity and specificity of indicators once again), floor/ceiling effects (the real law of initial values), reactivity (as defined earlier in this chapter), and skewness of data (which, unfortunately, is often ignored because of the easier usability of statistical methods that include the hypothesis that data are normally distributed). By summarizing these aspects, it can be concluded that ignoring the correlations between change and initial values leads to greater problems regarding aspects of reliability.

Several attempts have been made and suggestions have been published to control the correlations between change and initial values. An overview is given by Kallus (1997). Thereby the use of simple raw values after stimulation is the easiest method. Unfortunately, the influence of reactivity often leads to an increase in the variance of data and therefore an increase in beta errors. If there is no significant difference between groups with respect to an indicator, a process, or a diagnosis in the post-stimulus raw values, the significance may only ensue by correlation of the post-stimulus values with the basic values. This correlation can be easily made using the difference values. In this way the aforementioned flaws are taken into consideration but floor/ceiling effects are not. For the control of these well-known effects, so-called autonomic liability scores or an analysis of covariance can be used. These methods aim for a mathematical elimination of the variance that basic values have on the variance of change levels. These methods are prone to errors if the correlation between basic values and change values is not linear.

To overcome these methodological problems, the change itself can be analyzed. For this purpose, a so-called orthogonal polynomial analysis can be implemented. Thereby the change is divided into different components of trends. For example, a difference in the linear component occurs if one group shows in increase in an indicator during reaction whereas the other groups remain stable or show decreasing values. Differences in the quadratic component occur if one group shows a reaction like an inverse U-function whereas other groups remain stable or show linear changes. Nevertheless, these methods are prone to errors if there is no equidistance between the points of measurements.

However, each of these methods has strengths and weaknesses. Benjamin (1963) considered that there should be zero correlation between the initial level and a properly corrected score, and the adjusted score should have face validity. However, only scores calculated with the regression models will not be correlated with the initial level. Thus, for between-group comparisons, the analysis of covariance for the difference scores (D) adjusted for the initial level (X) is recommended (Benjamin, 1963). Individual differences in response to an experimental variable should be calculated as the difference from the covariance XD model, d − bDXx (Benjamin, 1963). Most methods are guided by the intention to control the correlation between change and initial values. They are created to yield at least clean change values. Nevertheless, the advantage of having mathematical control is offset by the disadvantage that information on reactivity is completely lost. If reactivity itself is the focus, a more qualitative approach is needed.

Qualitative Aspects of Reactivity

The use of a multidimensional multilevel approach should be considered as the most important paradigm with respect to qualitative aspects of reactivity. Aspects of psychometric techniques to measure changes should be integrated. In this context it should be recognized that correlations of indicators of different dimensions of human behavior are significant in most cases, but not substantial to declare the majority of variance is operationalized by simultaneous measurement of the indicators to receive more information by their change due to stimulation then only by looking for significant differences at the endpoint of measurement. For example, the investigation of activation in a specified setting should include not only self-ratings on activation but also measurement of heart rate, performance, and social aspects. Thus, it should be taken into consideration that every change in an indicator has to be separated from characteristic indicators of the baseline. For instance, a change in actual activation is influenced by the state of fatigue or other aspects of mood before the measurement. If somatic variables are measured, each actual change has to be correlated with illness or habitual handicaps of a person. For example, an increase in the heart rate in a person who has chronic heart disease needs an alternative interpretation compared with the same increase in a healthy person. In conclusion, baseline and change levels should be measured as specifically as possible. Last but not least, reactivity does not end with the protocol of measurement. Sometimes the processes of adaption, habituation, or regulation are also important for reaching the baseline.

If reactivity, therefore, is seen not only as a psychological phenomenon but as a psychophysiological one, the question about the interactions of these dimensions of human behavior arises. Specifically, it is of interest whether psychological aspects of behavior are able to denote variance in somatic indicators and vice versa. As can be seen in the next section, there is substantial evidence to accept this hypothesis. Data presented in Figures 6.3–6.6 were taken from Uhlig (2000) and modified for didactical reasons.

It is well-known that the induction of physical activity regularly leads to an increase in several somatic indicators such as heart rate, blood pressure, etc. The increase in the concentration of lactic acid is of particular interest

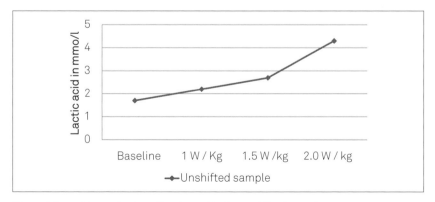

Figure 6.3   Concentration of lactic acid in the unshifted sample.

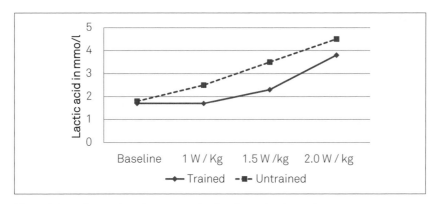

Figure 6.4   Comparison between trained and untrained samples.

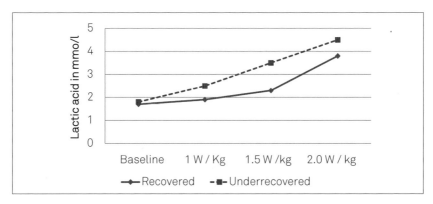

Figure 6.5   Comparison between recovered and under-recovered samples.

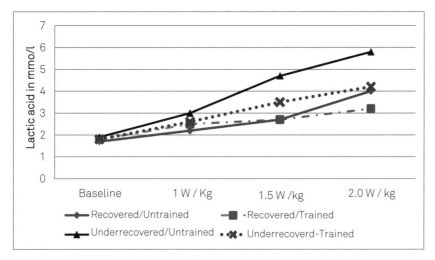

Figure 6.6   Concentration of lactic acid in different conditions.

because this indicator has a major impact on the diagnosis of fitness in humans. Higher levels of lactic acid under defined physical activity can be interpreted as a lower state of fitness compared with lower levels under the same workload. The increase in lactic acid is not linear but exponential, and if a level of 3–4 mmol/l is reached, the strength of activity is seen as critically high (Figure 6.3). Well-trained persons show lower levels of lactic acid than low-trained persons (Figure 6.4). If the increase in lactic acid under physical activity is seen not only as a result of a working musculature, but as a phenomenon of stress in general and the recovery–stress approach is used for differentiation between well-recovered and under-recovered persons, it can be hypothesized that there is also a difference between these two groups. Figure 6.5 leaves some evidence that this hypothesis can probably be accepted. And if, finally, the interaction between muscular fitness and state of recovery is addressed, it can be seen that the psychologically defined state of recovery is able to explain a valuable amount of variance in muscular fitness (Figure 6.6).

Final Considerations

More general, reactivity depends on the stimulus as well as the psychological and biological systems involved and also on the reaction itself, which should be analyzed regarding qualitative and quantitative aspects as well as the change itself. For practical reasons, it can be said that an environmental stimulus – whether psychological, biological, or social – is modified in any case by psychological, biological, or social factors. Well-known influencing factors are age, sex, the personality of a person, or – to put it in a more general context – every factor that can be considered as a shifting variable, able to explain the variance of a consecutive reaction of an individual. After that modification, the environmental stimulus mediates the final bio-psycho-social reaction. The mediators are different psychological, biological, or social systems with their own sensitivity, specificity, and therefore reactivity.

There is no doubt that dealing with reactivity in a psychological context is cumbersome and needs sophisticated methodology in research and practice. Nevertheless, this complexity should be accepted. Perhaps the steps forward are somewhat smaller in this context, but in the end the results are more precise and less prone to error.

References

Baethge, C. (2013). Nocebo: Die dunkle Seite der menschlichen Einbildungskraft [The dark side of human imagination]. *Deutsches Ärzteblatt, 110*(41), A-1904.

Benjamin, L.S. (1963). Statistical treatment of the Law of initial values (LAV) in autonomic research. A review and recommendations. *Psychosomatic Medicine, 25*(11–12), 556–566. https://doi.org/10.1097/00006842-196311000-00005

Burt, K.B., & Obradovic, J. (2013). The construct of psychophysiological reactivity. Statistical and psychometrical issues. *Developmental Review, 33*(1), 29–57. https://doi.org/10.1016/j.dr.2012.10.002

Chida, Y., & Steptoe, A. (2008). Cortisol awakening response and psychosocial factors: A review and meta-analysis. *Biological Psychology, 80*(3), 265–278. https://doi.org/10.1016/j.biopsycho.2008.10.004

Foerster, F., Schneider, H.-J., & Walschburger, P. (1983a). *Psychophysiologische Reaktionsmuster* [Psychophysiological reaction patterns]. Minerva.

Foerster, F., Schneider, H.-J., & Walschburger, P. (1983b). The differentiation of individual specificity, stimulus specificity and situational specificity response patterns in the activation process. *Biological Psychology, 17*(1), 1–26. https://doi.org/10.1016/j.biopsycho.2013.12.013

Franke, R.H., & Kaul, J.D. (1978). The Hawthorne experiments: First statistical interpretation. *American Sociological Review, 43*(5), 623–643.

Hinz, A., Hueber, B., Schreinicke, B., & Seibt, R. (2002). Temporal stability of psychophysiologic response patterns. Concepts and statistical tests. *Journal of Psychophysiology, 44*(1), 57–65. https://doi.org/10.1016/s0167-8760(01)00191-x

Jamieson, J. (1993). The law of initial values: Five factors or two. *Psychophysiology, 14*(3), 233–239. https://doi.org/10.1016/0167-8760(93)90037-P

Janke, W. (1974). Psychophysiologische Grundlagen des Verhaltens [Psychophysiological foundations of behavior]. In M. Kerekjarto (Ed.), *Medizinische Psychologie* (pp. 1–101). Springer. https://doi.org/10.1007/978-3-642-96203-5_1

Janke, W., & Kallus, K.W. (1995). Reaktivität [Reactivity]. In M. Amelang (Ed.), *Enzyklopädie der Psychologie* (Vol. C/VIII/2, pp. 1–89). Hogrefe.

Kallus, K.W. (1992). *Ausgangszustand und Beanspruchung* [Initial condition and stress]. Psychologie Verlags-Union.

Kallus, K.W. (1997). Indikatoren von Angst und Stress: Probleme der Reaktivität [Indicators of fear and stress: Problems of reactivity]. *Anästhesiologie-Intensivmedizin-Notfallmedizin-Schmerztherapie, 32*, 343–347. https://doi.org/10.1055/s-2007-995187

Uhlig, T. (2000). *Erholung als biopsychologisches Konstrukt* [Recreation as biological construct]. (Inaugural dissertation). Julius Maximilans Universität Würzburg.

Wilder, J. (1931). Das „Ausgangswert-Gesetz" – Ein unbeachtetes biologisches Gesetz und seine Bedeutung für Forschung und Praxis [Wilder's law of initial value]. *Klinische Wochenschrift, 10*, 1889–1893. https://doi.org/10.1007/BF01755704

Chapter 7
Recovery – The Forgotten Child in Human (Stress) Psychology

Thomas Uhlig and Christiane Uhlig

Abstract

Despite growing knowledge on stress and stress reactions, today it is not known to the same extent what happens in the organism to reach homeostasis again after exposure to stress. Recovery is needed to compensate for stress effects on the organism, to regain normal reactivity to cope adequately with subsequent taxing situations, and to allow the organism to consolidate adaptive processes by learning from stress and optimizing resources. Recovery is seen as a multilevel process in time for the re-establishment of bio-psycho-social resources and performance abilities. Following the description of the physiology and psychology of the stress response, this chapter describes different studies on how recovery evolves at the physical level. For human operators in various fields of aviation, the understanding of recovery is essential to ensure their tasks with cognitive performance while keeping the emotional impact low. Different notions such as coping, resilience and resource management, as well as regeneration and reparation are clarified.

Keywords: stress, recovery, psychophysiology

Introduction

Recently, new regulations were published requiring specific actions to ensure the management of stress and fatigue in operations. For example, the EU Regulation 2017/373 (2017), Annex 4, requests air traffic control service providers to prevent and mitigate the negative effects of stress and fatigue on air traffic controllers. It is further known from accident analyses that stressful situations lead to a variety of errors (Dismukes et al., 2018). Although there is growing knowledge on how stress and the stress reaction take place in humans, an open question remains: What happens in the organism to reach homeostasis again after the exposure to stress? One answer is given by the concept of coping. It is assumed that humans use (cognitive) strategies to cope with stressful stimuli and thereby are enabled to recover their psychophysiological reactions to stress. It is argued that a mismatch between the stress reaction and the coping process leads to underperformance, emotional dysfunction, and eventually to illness. Considering the empirical evidence, these are strong hypotheses. From the viewpoint of a broader approach, there are other hypotheses, too. From a biological point of view maintaining the homeostasis of an organism is a permanent process that is not only triggered by cognition. In addition, stress is not only a psychological phenomenon, but also a somatic one. The biological efforts of an organism to maintain homeostasis are described by terms such as reparation, regeneration, and recovery. In a recently published overview Kellmann and Beckmann (2018) reconfirmed the definition given by Kallus (2016) that, "recovery is a multilevel process in time for the re-establishment of bio-psycho-social resources and performance abilities" (Kallus, 2016, p. 53). These authors are established researchers in the field of recovery for more than 20 years. During that period the understanding of recovery as a challenging construct in psychology has been differentiated, elaborated, and partly redefined. Nevertheless, the basic considerations by Kellmann and Kallus (1999), Kellmann et al. (2001), and Uhlig (2000) are still present in the discussions.

In parallel, some alternative approaches are available in the current literature. These concepts enhance the understanding of recovery as one major element of humans' efforts to manage stressful situations. The question of whether these concepts have discriminative validity on their own or whether they should be considered as having a similar impact on the declaration of variance in data such as the stress–recovery approach is complex and puzzling. Nevertheless, in the field of applied psychology, as in work, sport, or aviation psychology, people have to deal with its complexity and may need basic remarks on the understanding of stress and recovery to establish a suitable frame for their work. This is the main purpose of this chapter.

Concepts and Definitions

On a meta-theoretical level, recovery includes a bundle of human efforts to stay stable in longer-lasting stressful situations and to manage these situations in an adequate manner including high (cognitive) performance and low (emotional) harm. Recognizing that the list is incomplete for constructs like regeneration and reparation, resilience or resource management is frequently used to express the feeling that humans are able to cover the effects of stress successfully. Since it is believed that these concepts differ in regard to aspects of stability over time and also in terms of the (bio-psycho-social) processes involved as the endpoints of a reaction or the goals that should be achieved, it is necessary to distinguish the concepts from one another. In this context, regeneration and reparation should be seen as various biological efforts and processes that are initiated if an anatomical structure or essential psychological process has been damaged. For example, sensorimotor functioning and cognitive performance are restored completely or only in part after a cerebral stroke. The efforts of the organism involved during this process of regeneration and reparation often remain unconscious. They are driven by somatic processes of healing and sometimes need support like pharmacological medication or psychotherapy.

By contrast, resilience and resource management are clearly defined psychological concepts and include the bio-psycho-social abilities of a person to avoid damage and to stay stable under stressful conditions. For example, in a study of 282 air traffic controllers, Schwarz et al. (2016) found effects of psychological stress on resilient behavior, but also a negative effect on safety culture development. These constructs should be considered as stable over time and play a major role in determining how a person reacts under stress. The term "recovery" is highly correlated with the basic principles of stress and the stress reaction in humans. Recovery is not passive but active, recovery may be correlated with coping, but has its own entity; recovery itself influences coping and vice versa. It can be hypothesized from these ideas that the role of recovery is underestimated as a substantial piece in the puzzle of stress. To our knowledge, no systematic review is available that integrates aspects of recovery into the concepts of human stress. No book is available in the psychological as well in the physiological or medical literature that is dedicated to recovery as a unique concept.

On the other hand, recovery is permanently present in everyday life. We take holidays for recovery (not for coping). We go to bed and sleep for the purpose of recovery (not for coping). We are active, eager for novel experiences, have fun, enjoy friendships, and much more for the purpose of recovery (not for coping). It cannot be denied that there is a common feeling of what recovery is. However, it cannot be said that there is a systematic evaluation about the question of what recovery really is. No doubt: Recovery is more than a feeling. It is an important piece of our life and an amazing concept that should be integrated into human (stress) psychology.

Stress in Humans

In an earlier time of stress research, these aspects were highlighted in the concepts by Cannon (1927) and Selye (1976). Cannon's introduction of the *fight-or-flight response* describes the physiological reactions that prepare an individual for the high efforts required to fight and run away. The fight-or-flight response is a species-typical response preparatory to fighting or fleeing, and is thought to be responsible for some of the deleterious effects of stressful situations on health. Selye's concept of the *general adaption syndrome* recognized that repeated responses to stressors can lead to harmful effects and longer-lasting effects on health. Both of these basic concepts have supplanted substantially cognitive and emotional aspects. The theory of James (1884) and Lange (1887), which claimed that behaviors and physiological responses are directly elicited by situations and that feelings of emotions are produced by feedback from these behaviors and responses, was elaborated by these paradigms and led to the understanding that aspects of perception can modulate the (emotional) response to a stressor. Lazarus and Folkman (1984) described the different efforts of individuals to avoid harmful effects of stressors on health and introduced aspects of coping into stress research. Newer concepts of stress and health psychology (Antonovsky, 1987) define aspects and effects of the stress response in the context of psychosocial resources that enable an individual to cope with stressors, whether adequate or not. Another approach is the introduction of aspects of recovery to describe individual resources as adequate (nonharmful) responses to stressors as a successful process of recovery to be responsible for a stable homeostasis.

Despite a tremendous number of data, most of the aforementioned concepts have not been introduced systematically as a framework for research and practice in applied psychology. As a consequence, there is a big lack of data, which makes it difficult to refer to a current opinion on stress and stress disorders in aviation psychology. Most of the papers published in this field focus only on some aspects of the bio-psycho-social stress response. Efforts have been made to introduce aspects of health-related quality of life (Eddleston et al., 2000) or posttraumatic stress disorder (PTSD; Stoll et al., 2000) into the paradigm of stress. In addition, emotional aspects of the stress response are discussed (Liu & Gropper, 2003) or the occurrence of acute and/or chronic cognitive dysfunction (Canet et al., 2003). Despite the impressive results reported in most of these papers, there is not enough empirical evidence for clear practical recommendations.

The question is: why? This is the leading question for the following remarks, which start with the physiology of the stress response.

Physiology of the Stress Response

The stress response involves autonomic, endocrine, and immune responses. The so-called stress hormones in acute stress response are epinephrine, norepinephrine, and steroid hormones such as glucocorticoids. The corticotropin-releasing hormone, a hormone stimulating the secretion of adrenocorticotropic hormone (ACTH) by the anterior pituitary gland, is also secreted in the brain. There, it elicits some of the emotional responses to stressful situations. Although increased levels of epinephrine and norepinephrine can raise blood pressure and heart rate, most of the harm to health comes from glucocorticoids. Prolonged exposure to high levels of these hormones can increase blood pressure, damage muscle tissue, lead to infertility, inhibit growth, inhibit the inflammatory response, and suppress the immune system.

In addition, there are multiple interrelations between the hypothalamo-pituitary axis (HPA) and neurotransmitter systems in the brain. The activity of the HPA is correlated with GABAergic, serotonergic, and dopaminergic responses, which are involved in psychiatric diseases and mood states like anxiety (GABAergic), depression (serotonergic), and psychosis (dopaminergic). On the other hand, HPA activity is believed to be involved in molecular processes of cell injury and/or tissue repair (Shipman et al., 2003) and therefore has direct influence on aspects of systemic inflammation, which plays a central role in intensive care medicine.

Nevertheless, there are still missing links between the psychophysiological aspects of the stress response and, for example, systemic inflammation.

Psychology of the Stress Response

The psychological aspects of the stress response include aspects of emotions and cognition. These aspects should be considered as moderator variables. They modify characteristics of the stressors and therefore influence the somatic stress response. For this reason, a cognitive evaluation of a stressor is of major interest. An interpretation of a stressor as harmful leads to negative emotions such as anxiety, fear, or depression. An interpretation of a stressor as challenging leads to positive emotions such as activation or joy. There is general consensus that stressor effects are either specific to the stressor itself, either for the individual who evaluates the stress or for the situation in which the stressor occurs. The impact of stressors on individual homeostasis is triggered in addition by the predictability of the stressor, the involvement of the individual, and the experience or ability of the individual to cope with stress. All these aspects are well elaborated in the psychological literature in general but not in the context of aviation psychology in particular. In addition, it is somewhat frustrating that most of the work on cognition and emotion in the context of stress is based on questionnaire-type measures. It would be helpful to receive systematic information about a person's stress history, but this approach is not used in daily practice.

Psychophysiology of the Stress Response

Biological responses to stress may be usefully examined at three levels, from perception of stress to short- and longer-term adaptive responses. It should be noted that any identified factor may be simultaneously stress promoting and stress relieving. This makes interpretation of research findings difficult, as frequently only the presence or absence of factors is described rather than what the presence or absence of a factor may represent to a particular subject. The mechanisms by which stressful events or circumstances produce psychological or somatic responses are complicated. The idea that the psychophysiological stress response should be discussed in terms of perception, immediate response, and a prolonged manifestation corresponds well to the biological principles that neurotransmitters can be distinguished on the basis of speed of response, duration of action, and range of activity. Inhibitory amino acids (e.g., GABA) and excitatory amino acids (e.g., glutamate) have specific, localized short-term effects. Monoamine transmitters (e.g., norepinephrine, dopamine), acetylcholine, and histamine produce slower but more durable responses that appear to modulate the actions of the primary amino acid transmitters. Neuropeptides (e.g., corticotropin-releasing factor and endorphins) produce even slower responses that tend to be more widespread and long lasting. Nevertheless, the discussions on the vulnerability to stress and the ability to cope with stressors should be elaborated. Beside stressful or adverse circumstances inducing symptoms or a disorder in an individual, another group of factors to consider are those influencing an individual's susceptibility to stress or their response to it. This leads to the discussion of aspects of coping and recovery.

Aspects of Coping and Recovery – The Recovery–Stress Approach

As mentioned in the previous sections, some of the harmful effects of stress are caused by the individual him-/herself. Some events that cause stress responses, such as prolonged exertion or extreme cold, cause damage directly. These stressors will affect everyone; their severity will depend on each person's physical capacity. The effects of other stressors, such as situations that cause fear or anxiety, depend on people's perceptions and emotional reactivity. That is, because of individual differences in temperament and experience with a particular situation, some people may find a situation stressful and others may not. In addition, the determination of whether a stressor is harmful or not is guided by the ability of the individual to control the stressor. Controlling the stressor and adequate reactivity in general are re-establishing the individual's homeostasis. This is called "coping."

An alternative to describe this process is the recovery–stress approach. The basic idea of a recovery–stress approach is that long-term negative effects of stressors occur if the organism is unable to unwind (Frankenhäuser, 1993), to restore resources, and to regain homeostatic and biorhythmic balance – in other words, to recover. The positive effects of recovery are at least threefold. First, stress effects are compensated; these may include changed hormonal status, changed metabolism, changed immune functioning, exhausted resources, cellular damage, changed thresholds in neurochemical functioning and neurochemical imbalance, as well as dysregulations in mood, action regulation, and social functioning. Second, the organism regains its normal reactivity, which allows it to cope adequately with subsequent taxing situations. Finally, recovery allows the organism to consolidate adaptive processes, thereby learning from stress and optimizing resources. Fitness and a high degree of competence and functioning will result from stress combined with optimal recovery. Increasing empirical evidence shows that recovery processes are impaired in individuals with a high risk of psychophysiological stress disorders (see Rau & Richter, 1994).

The recovery perspective changes the aspects of the current perspective on stress, stress mediators, and stress moderators in the following ways:

- Time window: According to a recovery–stress approach, reactions to stressful conditions should be monitored until a state of homeostatic balance has been re-established or new stressors occur, which could cause further disturbances of the individual.
- Systems: Stress research focuses on the aforementioned somatic systems and the central role of the HPA. The recovery–stress approach, by contrast, directs attention to those processes that compensate for the expenditure of resources, control excessive activation, and lead to the re-establishment of a homeostatic equilibrium and normal reactivity.
- Symptoms/indicators: Stress research focuses on negative psychological and somatic symptoms and how to reduce stress, while the recovery–stress state includes positive mood, well-being, life satisfaction, performance increments, the re-establishment and optimization of resources, and biological rhythms.

The recovery–stress perspective allows us to look at mediators and moderators of stress responses in an alternative way. For example, individuals are encouraged to seek social support, which offers social recovery. In the case of decision and action latitude (Karasek, 1993), individuals under stress are encouraged to create their own schedules and plan their own recovery activities and breaks. Recovery focuses on the (limited) resources of the individual. Resources can be divided into permanent resources and consumptive resources (Schönpflug, 1983). The resources concept allows us to define recovery as the re-establishment and optimization of resources after they have been taxed by stress due to challenges or threats to the individual. Dittmann, Kallus , and Van Damme (2000) contacted a study of European air traffic controllers on strain level resulting from stress and compensating recovery activities and found an association with situational and organizational conditions. To clarify the psychophysiological basis of the recovery-stress approach, some data are available to test the suitability of the stress–recovery approach in the field of acute medicine (Uhlig, 2016). These data include a categorization of patients depending on their psychosocial resources (e.g., state of chronic stress). It was shown that patients with a lower state of recovery reported higher levels of negative emotions and even pain during the perioperative period of open-heart surgery. In addition, those people showed a different reactivity of neurohumoral indicators of the stress response, which was represented in higher levels of renin and a dissociation of the HPA. Under-recovery was correlated with higher levels of ACTH and lower levels of cortisol during the perioperative period. In addition, those patients remained longer in the intensive care unit (ICU) and needed higher amounts of blood derivates.

The data on the reactivity of the HPA correspond well to the concept of overtraining in exercise physiology (Stein et al., 2002) and the concept of *chronic fatigue syndrome* in clinical psychology (Stein et al., 2002). In both fields a dissociation of the HPA is found to be the somatic equivalent of under-recovery with negative mood states being the psychological component.

Since some of these results are set in the framework of aspects on health-related quality of life or posttraumatic disorders, the question arises of whether the stress–recovery approach should be used as an additional concept with its own discriminative validity. This leads to discussions on PTSDs in the context of intensive care.

Posttraumatic Stress Disorders and Health-Related Quality of Life

The *Diagnostic and Statistical Manual of Mental Disorders* (DSM IV; American Psychiatric Association, 2000) describes PTSD as being caused by a situation in which a person experienced, witnessed, or was confronted with an event or events that involved actual or threatened death or serious injury, or a threat to the physical integrity of self or others (Cleare et al., 2001). As such, PTSD is a psychological disorder caused by exposure to a situation of extreme danger and stress. Symptoms include recurrent dreams or recollections, and can interfere with social activities as well as causing a feeling of hopelessness. The secondary phenomena include generalized anxiety, phobias, panic, hypervigilance, and agitation. A useful indicator of PTSD is how the individual has coped with previous loss or trauma in their life. People who have become intensely anxious or depressed following major life events may be particularly vulnerable.

It is not surprising that the somatic correlate of PTSD is once again the HPA. Outside the ICU, people with PTSD show lower levels of cortisol. It is hypothesized that a sensitization of ACTH receptors in the anterior pituitary gland in patients with PTSD decreases the secretion of cortisol in times of stress. Other studies show higher levels of corticotropin-releasing hormones in patients with PTSD compared with control individuals. It is obvious that PTSD impaired the health-related quality of life (HRQL). Data on the correlation between PTSD and HRQL show that a decline in HRQL is found in patients with symptoms of PTSD. In the context of elective open-heart surgery, a combination of high preoperative stress symptom scores, low aspects of HRQL, and high perioperative stress exposure with a longer duration of cardiopulmonary bypass were factors associated with adverse HRQL outcomes (Stoll et al., 2000).

From these data it is hypothesized, in addition, that the neurohumoral stress example, particularly the adrenergic and glucocorticoid response, are mediators for emotional and cognitive disorders. It is speculated that administration of stress hormones has dose-dependent effects on the incidence of symptoms of PTSD and therefore a decline in HRQL.

Of course, this hypothesis has psychological aspects, too. It is well known from psychopharmacology experiments that drug effects are modified by psychological variables such as factors of personality, coping styles, etc. (Buchanan & Lovallo, 2001; Schelling et al., 2003). Therefore, it is a suitable approach to consider drugs as research tools that show aspects of reactivity to stress and may elucidate the process of recovery if other variables such as severity of illness, type of surgery, age, and gender are considered, too.

Although it may be true that the longer the stress, the higher the decline in HRQL, it has to be examined whether time is the one and only factor in these effects. What about pain, fear, sleep, mobility etc.? All these factors are known to have substantial effects on the stress response and therefore on recovery.

Stress and stress disorders should therefore be integrated in a multidimensional multilevel approach considering psychological, somatic, and behavioral aspects. The stress response has to be considered as a process. The occurrence of stress disorders can be interpreted either as a consequence of acting humoral substances or as a result of failed recovery. Studies on the process of psycho-physiological recovery in the ICU are urgently warranted.

Aspects such as type of illness, age, and gender should be considered as factors influencing the stress response.

In addition, the interaction between molecular mechanisms of the healing process of tissues and the psycho-physiological stress response should be studied more intensively. The findings on the influence of chronic stress and a malfunction of the HPA on stress disorders are encouraging. Some of the results contribute to a concept that shows the importance of neurohumoral factors as a basis of psychological performance. This leads to conceptualization of *sickness behavior*.

Conceptualization of Sickness Behavior

Infection and inflammation often include behavioral aspects. Sick humans feel deactivated, weak, are not motivated for any activation, and show a lack of concentration. They show decreasing interest in their environment and they cut down eating and drinking. This constellation of unspecific symptoms of illness in general is called "sickness behavior" (Dantzer et al., 1993; Hart, 1988). Just as fever is described as a somatic reaction to infection and inflammation, sickness behavior is described in terms of behavioral changes that are reactions of an (infected) organism to cope with illness. Sickness behavior should be seen as an adaption to an infection that influences both the process of recovery and further illness. An inhibition of sickness behavior can lead to increasing morbidity and therefore mortality as documented for fever too (Hart, 1988). Although there are much fewer data on the importance of sickness behavior as necessary for survival, it is hypothesized that these behavioral changes are of similar importance. Nevertheless, there is much evidence that synchronization between metabolic, immunological, and behavioral symptoms of an infection depend on the same molecular signals as local immunological reactions. First of all, cytokines (interleukin [IL]-1, IL-6) and tumor necrosis factor alpha (TNF-alpha) are accused of playing a key role in the development of sickness behavior. Patients who received TNF-alpha as a therapeutic agent because of a viral infection or cancer showed symptoms of influenza in an early state of therapy and signs of depression and psychosis later on. Animals under cytokine treatment become anorectic and lethargic. Similar symptoms are found after an injection of lipopolysaccharide (LPS) (Kent et al., 1992; Krueger, 1990). Patients who receive IL-1 for therapy show sickness behavior every time after application (Schöbitz et al., 1994). There are multiple correlations between cytokines and behavior. These include aspects of fatigue and weakness, nausea and vomiting, eating disorders, sleeplessness, agitation, disorientation, hallucination, etc. This again makes it difficult to decide whether these symptoms shown by a patient are a consequence or the basis of an infection or a structural or other lesion. To elucidate the psycho-neuro-immunological aspects of behavior, some additional symptoms have to be discussed.

Fatigue

Fatigue is a common symptom in the general population as well as in patients. An important issue in the understanding of fatigue is the distinction between fatigue of short duration, which generally indicates a functional sign of the body that rest is required after effort, versus fatigue of prolonged duration, indicating a dysfunctional state in which rest does not restore energy but instead has a debilitating effect on functioning (Rubin & Hotopf, 2002). Fatigue is considered chronic when symptoms persist for at least 6 months. Fatigue is not the same as muscle weakness, depression, or muscle fatigability and it is not a nonspecific outcome of chronic illness (Chaudhuri & Behan, 2004). For clinical use, fatigue is best defined as difficulty in initiation or sustaining of voluntary activities. For postoperative fatigue it has been hypothesized that fatigue is a physiological response to surgery, with the assumption that the more severe the surgery, the more severe and prolonged the fatigue. A meta-analysis of studies on postoperative fatigue does not support this hypothesis (Hall & Salmon, 2002). There is strong evidence, albeit from a small study, for the hypothesis of an interrelation between fatigue and neurohumoral aspects. Considering fatigue as a part of the postoperative stress response, where the glucocorticoids and cytokines are dampened in particular (Rorarius et al., 2001), fatigue could be considered as a part of acute sickness behavior. For intensive care patients it has been shown that patients with sepsis who were randomized to receive corticosteroids did significantly better than those given placebo in terms of chronic fatigue and other neurobehavioral symptoms after recovery (Yehuda et al., 2002). Low cortisol concentrations predict development of PTSD after serious physical and psychological trauma. On the basis of neuroendocrine responses in fatigue disorders and a meta-analysis of 4,000 articles, Chaudhuri and Behan (2004) developed a biological model of central fatigue by which the key role of proinflammatory cytokines, the HPA axis, and the interrelation with peripheral adrenoceptors and corticoid receptors is shown. As in the case of sickness behavior – as a more global concept – it has to be argued for aspects of fatigue that despite increasing empirical evidence, no final recommendations can be given for practitioners. It remains open, for example, whether a person shows elevated levels of cytokines and therefore signs of inflammation because he or she is fatigued or whether he or she is fatigued because of the inflammation.

Aspects of Mood

Beyond all the studies of inflammation, sepsis, and the HPA axis, once again the interrelation between psychological aspects, in particular mood, the HPA axis, and cytokines, needs to be addressed. Since the seminal report by Besedowsky et al. (1986) that intraperitoneal injection of human IL-1β potentially activates the HPA axis in rats, the HPA-stimulating effects of IL-1 has been confirmed several times (Dunn, 2000). There seems to be general agreement that this response is a fundamental aspect of immune system communication with the nervous system. IL-6 and TNF-alpha share HPA-activating activity, although they are less potent and effective than IL-1. Since there is evidence that the rapid HPA-activating effects of IL-1 are impaired by COX inhibitors (Del Rey & Besedowsky, 1992), a strong correlation between the immune response and aspects of pain and analgesia can be confirmed. Another path of correlation comes from studies showing the HPA activation of IL-1 to be associated with increases in the apparent release of brain noradrenaline and serotonin (Wang & Dunn, 1998). Both the adrenergic and the serotonergic system are involved in behavioral aspects of activation and depression. Occurrence of these negative emotions could be blamed for higher rates of morbidity and mortality of patients (Kiecolt-Glaser et al., 2002). Thus not only the pathway from inflammation and the cytokines to the brain but also behavior should be discussed as responsible for an increased morbidity. Conversely, the way that the production of proinflammatory cytokines can be directly stimulated by negative emotions and stressful experiences should also be considered. Additionally, negative emotions also contribute to prolonged infection and delayed wound healing, processes that fuel sustained proinflammatory cytokine production. Recently the simultaneous involvement of negative emotions and life-threatening disease was considered for evaluating the relationship between anger and carotid artery arteriosclerosis (Bleil et al., 2004), depression and coronary artery disease (Appels et al., 2000), and hostility and coronary artery disease (Boyle et al., 2004). The results of these studies are supplemented by reports of the involvement of immunological markers (C-reactive protein, TNF-alpha) in the pathogenesis of the diseases (Cohen & Herbert, 1996; Jeanmonod et al., 2004; Suarez, 2004). The current opinion on aspects of mood and aspects of inflammation and disease can be summarized as follows (Cohen & Herbert, 1996):

1. There are plausible explanations of how psychological factors (like aspects of mood) might influence immunity and immune-mediated disease.
2. There is substantial evidence that psychological factors can influence both cellular and humoral indicators of immune status and function.
3. There are consistent and convincing reports of links between stress and disease onset and progression.

Cognitive Functions

Most of the aspects discussed in the previous section are strongly correlated with the occurrence of impaired cognitive functions. In a review, Gordon et al. (2004) give an overview of aspects of clinical identification of cognitive impairment. Although it is possible to identify cognitive impairment on the basis of objective (test scores) or subjective evidence, it remains undetected in most cases. Jackson et al. (2004) showed the importance of regular screening of persons for aspects of cognitive impairment. Thus, confounding factors like depression, pre-existing cognitive impairment, or any other medical diseases should be considered as mediators in particular. In addition, both of the reviews refer to the problem of statistical significance versus practical relevance of test scores. More studies are warranted that investigate the individual relevance of aspects of cognitive impairment in a specific context. From a more practical point of view, however, it is difficult to find an adequate neuropsychological test battery. Complete monitoring of cognitive functions is long lasting and cumbersome. Monitoring of only a few functions probably offers insufficient information for a correct diagnosis. By asking the question of which cognitive functions are important in aviation psychology, the research paradigm shifted to aspects of hippocampal (e.g., visual and verbal memory) and prefrontal cortex function (planning, organizing, self-monitoring abilities).

Conclusion

Dealing with questions about recovery in the context of aviation psychology first needs an answer of whether an impaired performance is the primary process or a secondary complication, for example, of systemic inflammation as a consequence of chronic stress. In addition, it has to be clarified whether the dysfunction is more structural or functional (agitation, confusion, cognitive dysfunction). Infection and inflammation often include behavioral aspects. Under-recovered persons feel deactivated, weak, are not motivated for any activation, and show a lack of concentration. They exhibit decreasing interest in their environment, and they eat and drink less. Aspects of sickness behavior are mediated in particular by cytokines. Nevertheless, it remains open whether a person shows elevated levels of cytokines and therefore signs of inflammation because he or she is fatigued, depressed, or dysphoric in general or whether he or she shows some of these symptoms because of inflammation.

References

American Psychiatric Association. (2000). *Diagnostic and statistical manual of mental disorders: DSM-IV-TR*. APA.

Antonovsky, A. (1987). *Unravelling the mystery of health. How people manage stress and stay well*. Jossey-Bass.

Appels, A., Bar, F.W., Bruggeman, C., & De Baets, M. (2000). Inflammation, depressive symptomatology, and coronary artery disease. *Psychosomatic Medicine, 62*, 601–605. https://doi.org/10.1097/00006842-200009000-00001

Besedowsky, H.O., Del Rey, A., Sorkin, E., & Dinarello, C.A. (1986). Immunoregulatory feedback between interleukin-1 and glucocorticoid hormones. *Science, 233*, 652–654. https://doi.org/10.1126/science.3014662

Bleil, M.E., McCaffery, J.M., Muldoon, M.F., Sutton-Tyrrell, K., & Manuck, S.B. (2004). Anger-related personality traits and carotid artery atherosclerosis in untreated hypertensive men. *Psychosomatic Medicine, 66*, 633–639. https://doi.org/10.1097/01.psy.0000138128.68838.50

Boyle, S.H., Williams, R.B., Mark, D.B., Brummett, B.H., Siegler, I.C., Helms, M.H., & Barefoot, J.C. (2004). Hostility as a predictor of survival in patients with coronary artery disease. *Psychosomatic Medicine, 66*, 629–632. https://doi.org/10.1097/01.psy.0000138122.93942.4a

Buchanan, T.W., & Lovallo, W.R. (2001). Enhanced memory for emotional material following stress-level cortisol treatment in humans. *Psychoneuroendocrinology, 26*, 307–317. https://doi.org/10.1016/s0306-4530(00)00058-5

Canet, J., Raeder, J., & Rasmussen, L.S., Enlund, M., Kuipers, H.M., Hanning, C.D., Jolles, J., Korttila, K., Siersma, V.D., Dodds, C., Abildstrom, H., Sneyd, J.R., Vila, P., Johnson, T., Muñoz Corsini, L., Silverstein, J.H., Nielsen, I.K., & Moller, J.T. (2003). Cognitive dysfunction after minor surgery in the elderly. *Acta Anaesthesiologica Scandinavica, 47*(10), 1204–1210. https://doi.org/10.1046/j.1399-6576.2003.00238.x

Cannon, W.B. (1927). The James-Lange theory of emotions: A critical examination and an alternative. *American Journal of Psychology, 39*, 106–124. https://doi.org/10.2307/1415404

Chaudhuri, A., & Behan, P.O. (2004). Fatigue in neurological disorders. *The Lancet, 363*, 978–988. https://doi.org/10.1016/S0140-6736(04)15794-2

Cleare, A.J., Blair, D., Chambers, S., & Wesseley, S. (2001). Urinary free cortisol in chronic fatigue syndrome. *American Journal of Psychiatry, 158*(4), 641–643. https://doi.org/10.1176/appi.ajp.158.4.641

Cohen, S., & Herbert, T.B. (1996). Health psychology: Psychological factors and physical disease from the perspective of human psychoneuroimmunology. *Annual Review of Psychology, 47*, 113–142. https://doi.org/10.1146/ANNUREV.PSYCH.47.1.113

Dantzer, R., Bluthe, R.M., Kent, S., & Goodall, G. (1993). Behavioral effects of cytokines: An insight into mechanisms of sickness behavior. In E. De Souza (Ed.), *Methods in neuroscience* (Vol. 17, pp. 130–149). Academic Press. https://doi.org/10.1016/S1043-9471(13)70013-2

Del Rey, A., & Besedowsky, H.O. (1992). Metabolic and neuroendocrine effects of proinflammatory cytokines. *European Journal of Clinical Investigation, Suppl. 1*, 10–15.

Dismukes, R. K., Kochan, J. A., & Goldsmith, T. E. (2018). Flight crew errors in challenging and stressful situations. *Aviation Psychology and Applied Human Factors, 8*(1), 25–46. https://doi.org/10.1027/2192-0923/a000129

Dittmann, A., & Kallus, K.-W., & Van Damme, D. (2000). *Integrated task and job analysis of air traffic controllers – Phase 3: Baseline reference of air traffic controller tasks and cognitive processes in the ECAC area.* EUROCONTROL.

Dunn, A. J. (2000). Cytokine activation of the HPA axis. *Annals of the New York Academy of Sciences, 917*, 608–615. https://doi.org/10.1111/j.1749-6632.2000.tb05426.x

Eddleston, J. M., White, P., & Guthrie, E. (2000). Survival, morbidity, and quality of life after discharge from intensive care. *Critical Care Medicine, 28*, 2293–2299. https://doi.org/10.1097/00003246-200007000-00018

EU Regulation 2017/373. (2017). *Requirements for providers of ATM/ANS and other ATM network functions and their oversight. Annex 4 Annex IV – Specific requirements for providers of air traffic services (Part-ATS).* http://eur-lex.europa.eu/legal-content/EN/TXT/PDF/?uri=CELEX:32017R0373&from=EN

Frankenhäuser, M. (1993). Psychoneuroendocrine approaches to the study of emotion as related to stress and coping. In H. E. Howe (Ed.), *Nebraska symposium on motivation* (pp. 123–161). University of Nebraska.

Gordon, M., Jackson, J. C., Ely, E. W., Burger, C., & Hopkins, R. O. (2004). Clinical identification of cognitive impairment in ICU survivors: Insights for intensivists. *Intensive Care Medicine, 30*, 1997–2008. https://doi.org/10.1007/s00134-004-2418-y

Hall, G., & Salmon, P. (2002). Physiological and psychological influences on postoperative fatigue. *Anesthesia & Analgesia, 95*(5), 1446–1450. https://doi.org/10.1097/00000539-200211000-00064

Hart, B. L. (1988). Biological basis of behaviour of sick animals. *Neuroscience & Biobehavioral Reviews, 12*(2), 123–127. https://doi.org/10.1016/s0149-7634(88)80004-6

Jackson, J. C., Gordon, S. M., Ely, E. W., Burger, C., & Hopkins, R. O. (2004). Research issues in the evaluation of cognitive impairment in intensive care unit survivors. *Intensive Care Medicine, 30*, 2009–2016. https://doi.org/10.1007/s00134-004-2422-2

James, W. (1884). What is an emotion? *Mind, 9*, 188–205. https://doi.org/10.1093/mind/os-IX.34.188

Jeanmonod, P., Kanel, R., Maly, F. E., & Fischer, J. E. (2004). Elevated plasma C-reactive protein in chronically distressed subjects who carry the a allele of the TNF-alpha-308 G/A polymorphism. *Psychosomatic Medicine, 66*, 501–506. https://doi.org/10.1097/01.psy.0000130903.78444.7d

Kallus, K. W. (2016). RESTQ-Basic: The general version of the RESTQ. In K. W. Kallus & M. Kellmann (Eds.), *The Recovery Stress Questionnaires. User manual* (pp. 49–85). Pearson Assessment.

Karasek, R. A. (1993). Job demands, job decision latitude and mental strain: Implications for job redesign. *Administrative Science Quarterly, 24*, 285–308. https://doi.org/10.2307/2392498

Kellmann, M., & Beckmann, J. (2018). *Sport, recovery and performance. Interdisciplinary insights.* Routledge. https://doi.org/10.4324/9781315268149

Kellmann, M., Altenburg, D., Lormes, W., & Steinacker, J. M. (2001). Assessing stress and recovery during preparation for the world championships in rowing. *Sport Psychologist, 15*, 151–167. https://doi.org/10.1123/tsp.15.2.151

Kellmann, M., & Kallus, K. W. (1999). Mood, recovery-stress state, and regeneration. In M. Lehmann, C. Foster, U. Gastmann, H. Keizer, & J. M. Steinacker (Eds.), *Overload, fatigue, performance incompetence, and regeneration in sport* (pp. 101–117). Plenum. https://doi.org/10.1007/978-0-585-34048-7_8

Kent, S., Bluthe, R. M., Kelley, K. W., & Dantzer, R. (1992). Sickness behavior as a new target for drug development. *Trends in Pharmacological Science, 13*, 24–29. https://doi.org/10.1016/0165-6147(92)90012-U

Kiecolt-Glaser, J. K., McGuire, L., Robles, T. F., & Glaser, R. (2002). Emotions, morbidity and mortality. *Annual Review of Psychology, 53*, 83–107. https://doi.org/10.1146/annurev.psych.53.100901.135217

Krueger, J. M. (1990). Somnogenic activity of immune response modifiers. *Trends in Pharmacological Sciences, 11*(3), 122–126. https://doi.org/10.1016/0165-6147(90)90198-H

Lange, C. G. (1887). *Über Gemütsbewegungen* [Considerations on changes of mood]. T. Thomas.

Lazarus, R. S., & Folkman, S. (1984). *Stress, appraisal, and coping.* Springer.

Liu, L. L., & Gropper, M. A. (2003). Postoperative analgesia and sedation in the adult intensive care unit. *Drugs, 63*(8), 755–767. https://doi.org/10.1016/0165-6147(90)90198-H

Rau, R., & Richter, P. (1994). *24-Stunden-Monitoring zur Prüfung der Reaktivität psychophysiologischer Parameter in Belastungs- und Erholungsphasen* [24-hours monitoring for assessing the reactivity of psychophysiological parameters in strain and recovery phases]. Forschungsbericht der Bundesanstalt für Arbeitsmedizin. Wirtschaftsverlag.

Rorarius, M. G. F., Kujansuu, E., Baer, G. A., Suominen, P., Teisala, K., Miettinnen, A., Ylitalo, P., & Laippala, P. (2001). Laparoscopically assisted vaginal and abdominal hysterectomy: comparison of postoperative pain, fatigue and systemic response. A case-control study. *European Journal of Anesthesiology, 18*, 530–539. https://doi.org/10.1016/0165-6147(90)90198-H

Rubin, G. J., & Hotopf, M. (2002). Systematic review and meta-analysis of interventions for postoperative fatigue. *British Journal of Surgery, 89*, 971–984. https://doi.org/10.1046/j.1365-2168.2002.02138.x

Schelling, G., Richter, M., Roozendaal, B., Rothenhäusler, H. B., Krauseneck, T., Stoll, C., Nollert, G., Schmidt, M., & Kapfhammer, H. P. (2003). Exposure to high stress in the intensive care unit may have negative effects on health-related quality-of-life outcomes after cardiac surgery. *Critical Care Medicine, 31*(7), 1971–1980. https://doi.org/10.1097/01.CCM.0000069512.10544.40

Schöbitz, B., de Kloet, E. R., & Holsboer, F. (1994). Cytokines in the healthy and diseased brain. *Physiology, 9*(3), 138–142. https://doi.org/10.1152/physiologyonline.1994.9.3.138

Schönpflug, W. (1983). Coping efficiency and situational demands. In R. Hockey (Ed.), *Stress and fatigue in human performance* (pp. 299–326). Wiley.

Schwarz, M., Kallus, K. W., & Gaisbachgrabner, K. (2016). Safety Culture, resilient behaviour, and stress in air traffic management. *Aviation Psychology and Applied Human Factors, 6*(1), 12–23. https://doi.org/10.1027/2192-0923/a000091

Selye, H. (1976). *The stress of life.* Mc Graw-Hill.

Shipman, J., Guy, J., & Abumrad, N. N. (2003). Repair of metabolic processes. *Critical Care Medicine, 31*(8), 512–518. https://doi.org/10.1027/2192-0923/a000091

Stein, M. B., Jang, K. L., Taylor, S., Vernon, P. A., & Livesley, W. J. (2002). Genetic and environmental influences on trauma exposure and posttraumatic stress disorder symptoms: A twin study. *American Journal of Psychiatry, 159*, 1675–1681. https://doi.org/10.1176/appi.ajp.159.10.1675

Stoll, C., Schelling, G., Goetz, A. E., Kilger, E., Bayer, A., Kapfhammer, H. P., Rothenhäusler, H. B., Kreuzer, E., Reichart, B., & Peter, K. (2000). Health-related quality of life and posttraumatic stress disorder in patients after cardiac surgery and intensive care treatment. *The Journal of Thoracic and Cardiovascular Surgery, 120*, 505–512. https://doi.org/10.1067/mtc.2000.108162

Suarez, E. (2004). C-Reactive protein is associated with psychological risk factors of cardiovascular disease in apparently healthy adults. *Psychosomatic Medicine, 66*, 684–691. https://doi.org/10.1097/01.psy.0000138281.73634.67

Uhlig, Th. (2016). The RESTQ-Risco. In K. W. Kallus & M. Kellmann (Eds.), *The Recovery Stress Questionnaires. User manual* (pp. 204–220). Pearson Assessment.

Uhlig, Th. (2000). *Erholung als biopsychologisches Konstrukt* (Inaugural Dissertation). Julius Maximilians Universität Würzburg.

Wang, J. P., & Dunn, A. J. (1998). Mouse interleukin-6 stimulates the HPA axis and increases brain tryptophan and serotonin metabolism. *Neurochemistry International, 33*, 143–154. https://doi.org/10.1016/s0197-0186(98)00016-3

Yehuda, R. (2002). Current status of cortisol findings in posttraumatic stress-disorder. *Psychiatric Clinics of North America, 25*, 341–368. https://doi.org/10.1016/s0193-953x(02)00002-3

Chapter 8
Analyzing Pilot Activity With Eye-Tracking Methods

Marie-Christine Bressolle, Gilles Devreux, Mauro Marchitto, and Thierry Baccino

Abstract

Different methods such as direct observation of users playing a flight scenario on a simulator, self-confrontation, semi-directive interviews, rating scales, etc. are generally used to assess human performance throughout a design cycle. In this chapter, we consider how to use physiological data such as eye fixations to bring additional evidence that could not be directly observed (or remembered by users). Although eye-tracking techniques are not new and were found to be valuable several decades ago, especially for laboratory settings, more recent advances in technology have led their use in the field of ecological evaluations. Recent head-mounted eye trackers can be used in natural interactions and multi-screen situations. The use of physiological data should, however, keep evolving in this field to help solve some difficulties in terms of data processing, validity, and usability. From this perspective, we describe the full setup of an eye-tracking study from calibration to data cleaning, selection of metrics, definition of areas of interest, and combined visualization with other contextual data. We offer insights into pupillometry, which is now commonly used for cognitive and emotional states assessment. Then, we open the discussion on how to include other physiological metrics such as heart rate variability, electrodermal activity, and body movement. This chapter aims to motivate further shared interests and developments in order to ease the use of physiological metrics, in addition to qualitative methods for assessing human performance in the cockpit.

Keywords: eye tracking, commercial aircraft, cockpit simulator, scanpath, pupil dilation, merged data, human factors

Introduction

The understanding of human cognitive performance, and of how pilots use new cockpit features in flight simulations, is a key challenge for cockpit design throughout the design cycle and ultimately for aviation safety. This chapter presents and discusses the interest in, the procedures, and the key methodological issues for applying eye tracking to cockpit design. Furthermore, classic human factors methods based on direct observation and on subjective outputs will be initially considered, together with their practical limitations. Whether collected during or after flight simulations, subjective outputs given by participants are widely used to understand their cognitive performance. They include both debriefing techniques and subjective rating scales. Subjective rating scales are often used for estimating experienced workload or situation awareness, for example,, the NASA task load index (TLX; Hart & Staveland, 1988), the modified Cooper–Harper scale (MCH; Casali & Wierwille, 1983), and the Situation Awareness Rating Technique (SART; Selcon & Taylor, 1990). In addition, the subjective outputs are also collected through debriefing sessions, or self-confrontation interviews, wherein participants describe their perception, understanding, or intentions. Their relevance rests on respondents' ability to remember the details of the course of actions. Consequently, they cannot properly address behaviors that are automatic and unconscious, such as eye movements, to inform explicitly about attended information. Moreover, there might be subjective response biases. Finally, *online* ratings (i.e., collected while piloting) might be intrusive, as there could be an interference with the pilot's primary task.

Performance measures and observational data of participants' behavior provide further fruitful outputs for understanding human performance. However, these observations also fail to capture many behavior details. Therefore, the need for more objective measures is of importance. The visual behavior recorded during a simulated session helps to understand underlying cognitive activities. The replay of the gaze video can also be used later for self-confrontation during debriefing sessions. Similarly, physiological parameters, such as heart rate and pupil diameter, can be analyzed to better understand pilots' effort and performance.

Eye-tracking measures have existed for several decades, but only recently have they become feasible for recording in ecological situations. A key step in the eye-tracking history was made in 1947 when Paul Fitts and his colleagues (Fitts et al., Jones, & Milton, 1950) used motion picture cameras to study the movements of pilots' eyes while they used cockpit controls and instruments to land an airplane. Jacob and Karn (2003), considered the study of Fitts to be the earliest application of eye tracking to usability engineering (i.e., the systematic study of users interacting with products to improve product design). Eye tracking flourished in the 1970s, showing great advances in both tracking technology and psychological theory to link eye-tracking data to cognitive processes (Jacob & Karn, 2003). Most recent eye-tracking devices are fairly reliable, minimally invasive, and easy to operate, with some tracked data being available in real time. All these improvements enable the integration of eye trackers in ecological situations for cockpit evaluation.

Several studies show that recent eye-tracking devices provide valuable data for investigating pilots' visual behaviors and cognitive performance in order to improve cockpit designs (Dehais et al., 2010; Moacdieh et al., 2013; for a review, see Peißl et al., 2018). For Li et al. (2015), the visual scan pattern is one of the most powerful metrics for assessing a pilot's cognitive processes in the cockpit, such as attention shifts while performing tasks. The use of eye tracking can support the system design team in understanding pilots' attention distribution, situational awareness, and perceived workload.

Although eye-tracking techniques are widely recognized as offering valuable data, several key issues need to be considered to ensure valid data collection and analysis (Li et al., 2015). This chapter aims to discuss important aspects to extend the introduction of eye tracking and further improve human tracking in cockpit design processes, from evaluation set-up to metrics selection and data analysis.

Firstly, depending on the nature of the tasks, the choice to be made is still between a remote eye-tracking system with some restrictions on the participant's head movement or a head-mounted system that could impact the participant's comfort and introduce restrictions in the field of view. Thus, to acquire robust eye movement data and establish a relationship with the area of interest (AOI) in the scene, another key issue is accuracy, which still remains a challenge in ecological situations. The selection of proper eye movement metrics also has to be considered: fixations (during which visual information is acquired), saccades (change of visual focus location), pupil diameter, or other parameters. Selected indicators must fulfill the objectives of the evaluation: Examples might be the lapse of time after an event during which participants do not glance at AOIs, the dwell time on specific AOIs, the number of fixations, or the visual scan sequence during selected periods of the simulation. Similarly, the interpretation of metrics should be considered (e.g., the dwell time indicating more time spent on interpreting or processing the information; pupil dilation related to higher mental workload). In addition to quantitative outputs (e.g., dwell time on main AOI), we highlight the benefit of performing individual eye-tracking qualitative analyses to gain a deeper understanding of visual strategies on specific AOIs. We also highlight the advantage of using gaze video in debriefing sessions as a powerful means for collecting verbal outputs from participants (such as reported difficulties or explanations for a better understanding of their visual strategies and performance). Here, we discuss the need to develop further adapted metrics (e.g., similarity) and processing capabilities to increase coverage and usability of eye-tracking data collection and analysis. Finally, we introduce the perspective of combining eye tracking with other physiological data such as heart rate variation for workload assessment and motion capture for the assessment of a pilot's posture and movements.

Eye-Tracking Set-Up in a Cockpit Simulator

Psychophysiological measures, including visual behavior data (e.g., a pilot's visual scanning on available data or attention allocation on a particular display), offer the possibility of recording objective data of participants while they perform a task and of better evaluating interactions with new cockpit features. The experimental protocols that include the three categories of measures such as the participants' verbal exposure, the experimenters' observations and records, and physiological data such as eye movement parameters (e.g., eye fixations, pupil diameter variation) lend higher reliability to the results generated. Depending on the objectives of the evaluations, the first approach is to compare situations where the new design features were introduced versus situations not including these features in order to understand how they impacted performance. A second complementary approach is to examine how participants used particular information while recording their performance and subjective outputs.

In the context of cockpit evaluations, recent portable eye trackers have the advantage of being easily moved and used on the different simulators with low constraints imposed on the participants' freedom of movement. Although their usability (e.g., in terms of calibration duration) is still not fully optimal or equivalent, many wearable devices can be used for cockpit evaluation.

Since the eye tracker system does not provide 100 % accuracy, some criticisms have arisen regarding the relevance of the eye-tracking data gathered. With some precautions, these data are still relevant in the context of applied studies. First, depending on the eye-tracker accuracy and the distance of the eye to the AOI, the smallest acceptable AOI size can be computed. For example, 1° (degree of visual angle) corresponds to 1 cm at an observation distance of approximately 57 cm (Scharff, 2003). In the case of an eye tracker accuracy of 0.5° (i.e., a potential measurement error of 0.5° from the detected gaze point) and a pilot looking at a display at a distance of

57 cm, the smallest acceptable AOI would be a circle with radius of $r = 0.5$ cm. In this specific context, we classified three types of AOI depending on their sizes: large AOI, (e.g., full display such as navigational display [ND] and primary flight display [PFD] or a larger area such as the windshield), medium AOI (e.g., the major elements of the PFD such as speed scale, heading scale, etc.), and small AOI (e.g., the dynamic elements on the ND and PFD such as flight director, flight path vector, etc.). Second, AOI ecological contextualization can be done by integrating other sources of data during the analysis such as: observations, data recorded on pilots' actions and flight scenario events, and pilots' verbalizations collected during the session and during debriefings. The video of the gaze position can also be used in a debriefing session as a means of auto-confrontation.

Relevant Eye-Tracking Metrics

This section presents examples of metrics used as indicators for questions related to the introduction of new cockpit features such as assessing their impact on pilots' gaze repartition (e.g., head-up vs. head-down), visual pattern (e.g., scanning of the cockpit displays), and mental workload.

Eye movements are typically divided into fixations and saccades: Fixation is the moment when the eyes are relatively stationary, taking in or encoding information, and saccade is an eye movement occurring between fixations, typically lasting 10–35 ms. The purpose of most saccades is to move the eyes to the next viewing position. Most information from the eye is made available during a fixation but not during a saccade due to the saccadic suppression phenomenon (Gregory, 1990). In fact, saccades are ballistic movements (meaning that it is nearly impossible to modify their speed, amplitude, or direction once the movement has started), whose parameters are coded in the central nervous system before specific motor neurons realize the movement. The saccadic suppression phenomenon prevents large changes in object location within the visual scene being detected by the brain (Bridgeman et al., 1975). Eye-movement metrics may be classified as *synchronic* indicators such as fixation (duration, number, etc.) or saccade (amplitude, velocity, etc.) and *diachronic* indicators (scanpaths or saliency maps). Synchronic means that an event occurs at a specific point in time and possibly in a specific AOI, while diachronic means that this event is taken into account over time (Le Meur & Baccino, 2013).

According to Table 8.1, one alternative classification is to consider the type of processing involved by these metrics. Generally, time metrics reflect ongoing cognitive processes (e.g., understanding) while space metrics are dedicated to spatial strategies and allocation of attention. Most eye-tracking studies in ergonomics (Kilingaru et al., 2013; Marchitto et al., 2016; Sirevaag et al., 1999; Tole et al., 1982; Van De Merwe et al., 2012; see also Peißl et al., 2018, for a review) have heavily used cumulative fixation time and AOI approaches, dividing a visual scene into predefined AOI. Transitions into and from these areas, as well as time spent in each area, are tallied.

Table 8.1 Examples of metrics for synchronic and diachronic analysis

Metrics	Synchronic Analysis	Diachronic Analysis
Time	• Dwell Time (ms) • Entry Time (ms) • Refixations (N and ms)	• Scanpaths Similarity (Levensthein distance ...) • Transition Matrix
Space	• Saccade Amplitude (mm/pix) • Gaze position distribution (%)	
Others	• Pupil diameter	• Pupillometry: TERPs (Task-Evoked Pupillary Responses) • Blink Frequency

The dwell time can be used as a global measure including all pilots' sample data. This metric was used, for instance, as an indicator of pilots' gaze repartition between head-up (outside of the windshield) and head-down position (on PFD and ND). Comparing two situations (reference situation and situation with new feature), this approach offers an objective output on how the attention repartition was impacted (and divided between AOIs) for a sample of pilots.

A deeper understanding of cognitive performance needs to be complemented by an individual analysis regarding the pilot's scanpath, such as materialized by AOI sequence charts. While the previous approach can signal areas where more or less attention is spent, few investigations have considered the complex nature of scanpaths, defined from a series of fixations and saccades on the scene. For this purpose, the AOI sequence chart, basically a chronogram with AOI entry times and visit durations dependent on time, can be used as a means of visualization. The AOI sequence also constitutes a basis for a multisource representation of data. After data synchronization, which is essential to align recorded simulator data (a pilot's actions, aircraft state data such as flight level, distance from runway, etc., and scenario events such as failures, weather, etc.) to the pilot's psychophysiological data, we can superpose relevant information such as flight profile and key scenario events to eye-tracking data.

Figure 8.1 represents a chronogram of a pilot's scanning pattern during a flight scenario after an erroneous altitude display on PFD (called "failure" in Figure 8.1). The scanning pattern represented on the sequence chart high-

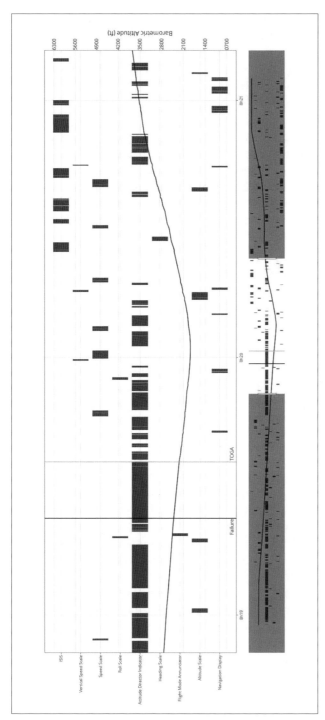

Figure 8.1   Example of an area of interest sequence time (ms) representing a scanning pattern following a scripted failure, according to the altitude (ft) and the scenario time TOGA = Takeoff/Go-Around; ISIS = integrated standby instrument system.

lights what display was used by the pilot (e.g., the integrated standby instrument system [ISIS] backup display after engaging the go-around procedure). During the failure, the pilot focused on the attitude director indicator (ADI); after the failure alarm, the scan path scattered across the instruments, to focus finally on the ISIS. The pilot's verbalizations confirmed that the pilot initiated TOGA (Takeoff/Go-Around) right after the alarm but had to go through various instruments to better understand the situation and improve his awareness and then use the backup system as a primary source of information.

The graph was drawn using the R libraries ggplot2 and plotly (Plotly Inc., 2015; Wickham, 2016). The idea is to allocate a y-coordinate to each AOI and add the following geoms (i.e., geometric objects of ggplot2):

1. Rectangles geom with event start (beginning of the fixation) as origin point on the x-axis and fixations durations as rectangle length;
2. Line geom for the flight levels data (depending on the difference of recording frequencies between the eye-tracking system and the simulator, an interpolation might improve the visual rendition); and
3. Vertical lines geom for discrete scenario events.

One issue that can be encountered with this type of visualization is the overdensity of the data for lengthy scenarios. Two methods can be used to mitigate it, allowing the specialist to dig through the data:

1. Create a plot array with predefined periods of interest (e.g., for the approach phase); and
2. Use the scanning and panning function of Plotly to scroll through the graph.

This method can be scripted for automation purpose using any appropriate language. A dedicated graphical user interface can be developed to improve the ease of use and to create powerful visualizations.

After an individual analysis, an open question is to obtain a global picture for the whole sample of pilots.

Several metrics have been devised to compare scanpaths (Le Meur & Baccino, 2013), using either distance-based methods (string edit technique or Levenshtein distance) or vector-based methods. Distance-based methods compare scanpaths only from their spatial characteristics, while vector-based approaches allow for comparison across different dimensions (frequency, time, etc.). The representation of string edit distance can take the form of a matrix showing the score for every comparison. This metric can provide a numerical value of the difference between an expected and an actual behavior, between pilots (with a carefully controlled experimental situation), or between different instances of the same function. Using this method, we should be able to highlight extreme statistical units worth investigating.

Pupillometry is interesting mostly for tracking emotional processes (e.g., fear, happiness; Guillot et al., 2014) or attentional workload (Ahlstrom & Friedman-Berg, 2006; Beatty, 1982). Pupil diameter represents raw data provided as samples (in sample frequency) and values are typically given in pixels of the eye camera or in millimeters. It is easier to use the horizontal diameter because the vertical diameter is too sensitive to eyelid closures. When using pupil diameter as a measure of cognitive or emotional states, it is important to remember that the cognitive and emotional effects on pupil diameter are small and easily drown in the large changes due to variation in light intensity. Varying brightness of the stimulus (screen) may therefore introduce artifacts into the data. In human factors studies with participants in situations with a natural variation in luminance, for instance, airplane pilots or when using web pages for stimuli, it is particularly difficult to analyze pupil diameter if luminance is not constant. Algorithms that compensate for changes in luminance have appeared, which analyze the variation in light on the stimulus monitor, using wavelets (Marshall, 2007; Pedrotti et al., 2014) or blind source separation techniques (BSS) such as principal component analysis (PCA; Oliveira et al., 2009) or independent component analysis (ICA; Jainta & Baccino, 2010). The principle of BSS is the separation of a set of signals from a set of mixed signals, without the aid of any information (or with little information) about the source signals or the mixing process. BSS methods have proven their usefulness in identifying the signal of cognitive load in pupillary responses (Jainta &and Baccino, 2010). However, these algorithms do not consider the level of luminance, they only try to separate different processes. We believe a better way is to record the luminance intensity concurrently with pupil diameter and eliminate the luminance effect using the Watson formula (Watson & Yellott, 2012). These authors developed a mathematical function incorporating several parameters of the pupil (luminance, field size of the adapting field, age of the observer, etc.) that predict a mean pupil diameter (PD). Of course, this mean PD may be different than the observed PD since considerable variability may occur in real life mainly due to endogenous stimuli.

In the human factors area, PD is one in a family of measures used to examine mental workload and cognitive processing. PD is often combined with blink rate and duration, fixation durations, saccadic extent, fixation rate, and dwell time, to estimate the cognitive requirements of different tasks (Brookings et al., 1996; Van Orden et al., 2000). While blink rate, blink duration, and fixation duration all tend to decline as a function of increased workload (Van Orden et al., 2000; Veltman & Gaillard, 1998), pupil dilation instead increases (Iqbal et al., 2004; Van Orden et al., 2000). Van Gerven et al. (2004) found that mean pupil dilation is a useful event-related measure of cognitive load in research on education and learning.

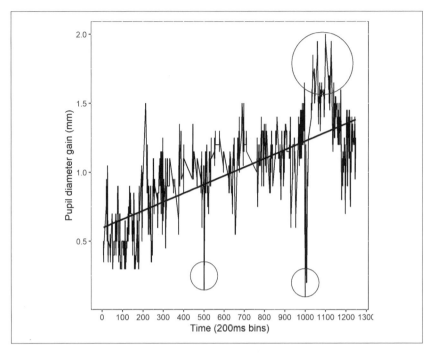

Figure 8.2   Pupil diameter variation for one pilot as a function of time (bins, 200 ms) with significant peaks identifying potential cognitive workload.

As an illustration of this method, Figure 8.2 shows the gain variation for one representative pilot for the main AOIs as a function of time bins.

In practice, three major steps were drawn to use this method:

1. The values of the two pupils' size are averaged, and only a mean pupil size is considered. Data are resampled in bins of 200 ms (pupil reaction time) and then arranged as a function of time and AOIs.
2. After having calculated the theoretical PD (Watson's formula), the mean PD is then subtracted from observed (recorded) PD values to obtain a distribution of pupil size changes free of any luminance variation. The only remaining variations are due to endogenous phenomena.
3. In order to extract the most significant peaks of PD, a regression analysis with time as predictor and pupil size as criterion allows for the computation of residual values.

Here the bins around 500 show extreme negative residual values that reflect a significant constriction (miosis) of the pupil, while the bins around 1,100 show extreme positive residual values that reflect a significant dilation (mydriasis) of the pupil. The effect occurring during this last period could be explained by a subsequent failure. Although in this case the observed phenomenon seems to be event-related, we believe that this method could potentially allow us to highlight the unexpected workload generation due to the design effect. But in order to reinforce the detection of such effect, a multisource analysis should be conducted. The next section discussed the benefit and challenges of adding other sources of data for workload assessment.

Perspectives: Combining Eye Tracking With Other Physiological Devices

This section presents the coupling of eye-tracking recording to other psychophysiological markers of cognitive activity, that is, electrocardiogram (ECG) and electrodermal activity (EDA), and to the body's motion capture data (MoCap), to monitor body posture and movements. The issue of recording system synchronization is also addressed. Being multidimensional as a construct, workload can be inferred from various sources (Leplat, 1978; Parasuraman et al., 2008; Wierwille & Eggemeier, 1993). The methodology for analyzing and interpreting the cardiac and electrodermal activity is presented in Chapter 9 by Koglbauer and Braunstingl (2021) in this volume.

As for MoCap, it is typically required to wear reflective markers on specific body locations that are mapped by infrared cameras installed within the cockpit simulator, and previously calibrated. The system records the tridimensional position and rotation of markers (with respect to a predefined origin), couples them with a previously created body model (body calibration phase), and infers the position of body articulations. Variations in each body segment position, and the *travelled distance* within a specific time period, are then computed. It was shown recently that body movements give reliable markers of cognitive engagement (Kaakinen et al., 2018): In this study, it was found that during reading of task-relevant text segments, the head-to-screen distance and speed of head motion (participants were reading on a tablet) decreased as compared with when reading task-irrelevant text segments. This variation of distance/speed has been interpreted to indicate a dynamic engagement that expresses the way readers have embodied the demands of cognitive tasks during the reading process.

For synchronization purposes, the eye tracker, psychophysiological device, and MoCap should be connected to a common relay box and a dedicated software able to generate marker signals (e.g., a 5-V input) that would be recorded by the three systems in parallel. Synchronization between the recorded data and the simulator (i.e., operational context) can be performed offline. One option is to create a marker that could be easily recognized in the simulator log file and in at least one recording system. For example, to switch on an LED light with an associated sound (e.g., autopilot button) while looking at it allows the scene camera integrated in the eye-tracking glasses to capture such moments, which are also recorded in the simulator log file.

Specific software also exists enabling the synchronization of files for overall data visualization. Although synchronization issues might be resolved by means of recording of digital markers, this software may help in filtering the results on the basis of multiple criteria, before computing basic metrics for statistical analysis (e.g., to analyze HR only during a specific flight period, based on an aircraft parameter).

Conclusion

By using eye-tracking devices in combination with other existing techniques (observation, rating scales, etc.), design teams can evaluate the visual behavior of pilots on cockpit interfaces to assess usability and cognitive performance. Multiple current studies use eye-tracking devices to investigate pilot visual behaviors and facilitate the system design team's understanding of pilots' cognitive performance (attention distribution, workload, etc., cf. Peißl et al., 2018, for a review). Such objective data provide valuable input for improvements in cockpit design through a human-centered design process. Moreover, recent advances in eye-tracking technology make it possible to introduce eye-tracker devices in ecological situations with a reasonable impact (e.g., on pilots' comfort, field of view, etc.) keeping the balance in favor of using such devices. However, as discussed in this chapter, it is still necessary to consider certain key methodological issues (e.g., individual analysis, similarity analysis) and some required overall usability improvements (e.g., data analysis procedures and tools) to extend the use of such technologies for ecological evaluations in an industrial context in an iterative design process. This chapter makes concrete suggestions to support a step toward this direction.

References

Ahlstrom, U., & Friedman-Berg, F. J. (2006). Using eye movement activity as a correlate of cognitive workload. *International Journal of Industrial Ergonomics, 36*(7), 623–636. https://doi.org/10.1016/j.ergon.2006.04.002

Beatty, J. (1982). Task-evoked pupillary responses, processing load, and the structure of processing resources. *Psychological Bulletin, 91*(2), 276. https://doi.org/10.1037/0033-2909.91.2.276

Bridgeman, B., Hendry, D., & Stark, L. (1975). Failure to detect displacement of the visual world during saccadic eye movements. *Vision Research, 15*(6), 719–722. https://doi.org/10.1016/0042-6989(75)90290-4

Brookings, J. B., Wilson, G. F., & Swain, C. R. (1996). Psychophysiological responses to changes in workload during simulated air traffic control. *Biological Psychology, 42*(3), 361–377. https://doi.org/10.1016/0301-0511(95)05167-8

Casali, J. G., & Wierwille, W. W. (1983). A comparison of rating scale, secondary-task, physiological, and primary-task workload estimation techniques in a simulated flight task emphasizing communications load. *Human Factors, 25*(6), 623–641. https://doi.org/10.1177/001872088302500602

Dehais, F., Tessier, C., Christophe, L., & Reuzeau, F. (2010). The perseveration syndrome in the pilot's activity: Guidelines and cognitive countermeasures. *Lecture Notes in Computer Science, 5962*, 68–80. https://doi.org/10.1007/978-3-642-11750-3_6

Fitts, P. M., Jones, R. E., & Milton, J. L. (1950). Eye movements of aircraft pilots during instrument-landing approaches. *Aeronautical Engineering Review, 9*(2), 24–29.

Gregory, R. L. (1990). *Eye and brain* (4th ed.). Weidenfeld and Nicolson.

Guillot, G., Courcoux, P., Garrel, C., Baccino, T., & Schlich, P. (2014). Pupillometry of taste: Methodological guide–from acquisition to data processing–and toolbox for MATLAB. *The Quantitative Methods for Psychology, 2*(10), 179–195. https://doi.org/10.20982/tqmp.10.2.p179

Hart, S. G., & Staveland, L. E. (1988). Development of NASA-TLX (Task Load Index): Results of empirical and theoretical research. *Advances in Psychology, 52*, 139–183. https://doi.org/10.1016/S0166-4115(08)62386-9

Iqbal, S. T., Zheng, X. S., & Bailey, B. P. (2004, April). Task-evoked pupillary response to mental workload in human-computer interaction. In ACM (Ed.), *CHI'04 extended abstracts on human factors in computing systems* (pp. 1477–1480). ACM. https://doi.org/10.1145/985921.986094

Jacob, R. J. K., & Karn, K. S. (2003). Eye tracking in human-computer interaction and usability research. ready to deliver the promises. In J. Hyönä, R. Radach, & H. Deubel (Eds.), *The mind's eye: Cognitive and applied aspects of eye movement research* (pp. 531–553). https://doi.org/10.1016/B978-044451020-4/50031-1

Jainta, S., & Baccino, T. (2010). Analyzing the pupil response due to increased cognitive demand: An independent component analysis study. *International Journal of Psychophysiology, 77*, 1–7. https://doi.org/10.1016/j.ijpsycho.2010.03.008

Kaakinen, J. K., Ballenghein, U., Tissier, G., & Baccino, T. (2018). Fluctuation in cognitive engagement during reading: Evidence from concurrent recordings of postural and eye movements. *Journal of Experimental Psychology: Learning, Memory, and Cognition, 44*(10), 1671. https://doi.org/10.1037/xlm0000539

Kilingaru, K., Tweedale, J. W., Thatcher, S., & Jain, L. C. (2013). Monitoring pilot "situation awareness". *Journal of Intelligent & Fuzzy Systems, 24*(3), 457–466. https://doi.org/10.3233/IFS-2012-0566

Koglbauer, I. V., & Braunstingl, R. (2021). Applications of Cardiac and Electrodermal Activity Assessment in Aviation. In I. V. Koglbauer, & S. Biede-Straussberger (Eds.), *Aviation Psychology: Applied Methods and Techniques* (pp. 141–162). Hogrefe.

Le Meur, O., & Baccino, T. (2013). Methods for comparing scanpaths and saliency maps: strengths and weaknesses. *Behavior Research Methods, 45*(1), 251–266. https://doi.org/10.3758_s13428-012-0226-9

Leplat, J. (1978). The factors affecting workload. *Ergonomics, 21*, 143–149. https://doi.org/10.1080/00140137808931709

Li, W. C., Yu, C. S., Greaves, M., & Braithwaite, G. (2015). How cockpit design impacts pilots' attention distribution and perceived workload during aiming a stationary target. *Procedia Manufacturing, 3*(AHFE), 5663–5669. https://doi.org/10.1016/j.promfg.2015.07.781

Marchitto, M., Benedetto, S., Baccino, T., & Cañas, J. J. (2016). Air traffic control: Ocular metrics reflect cognitive complexity. *International Journal of Industrial Ergonomics, 54*, 120–130. https://doi.org/10.1016/j.ergon.2016.05.010

Marshall, S. P. (2007). Identifying cognitive state from eye metrics. *Aviation, Space, and Environmental Medicine, 78*(5), B165–B175.

Moacdieh, N. M., Prinet, J. C., & Sarter, N. B. (2013). Effects of modern primary flight display clutter: Evidence from performance and eye tracking data. *Proceedings of the Human Factors and Ergonomics Society, 1*, 11–15. https://doi.org/10.1177/1541931213571005

Oliveira, F. T., Aula, A., & Russell, D. M. (2009). Discriminating the relevance of web search results with measures of pupil size. In ACM (Ed.), *Proceedings of the SIGCHI Conference on Human Factors in Computing Systems* (pp. 2209–2212). ACM. https://doi.org/10.1145/1518701.1519038

Parasuraman, R., Sheridan, T. B., & Wickens, C. D. (2008). Situation awareness, mental workload, and trust in automation: Viable, empirically supported cognitive engineering constructs. *Journal of Cognitive Engineering and Decision Making, 2*(2), 140–160.

Pedrotti, M., Mirzaei, M. A., Tedesco, A., Chardonnet, J.-R., Mérienne, F., Benedetto, S., & Baccino, T. (2014). Automatic stress classification with pupil diameter analysis. *International Journal of Human-Computer Interaction, 30*(3), 220–236. https://doi.org/10.1080/10447318.2013.848320

Peißl, S., Wickens, C. D., & Baruah, R. (2018). Eye-tracking measures in aviation: A selective literature review. *The International Journal of Aerospace Psychology, 28*(3–4), 98–112. https://doi.org/10.1080/24721840.2018.Peis1514978

Plotly. (2015). *Collaborative data science.* Plotly Technologies Inc. https://plot.ly

Scharff, L. F. V. (2003). Sensation and perception research methods. In S. F. Davis (Ed.), *Handbook of Research Methods in Experimental Psychology* (Vol. 263, pp. 263–284). Blackwell Publishing Ltd.

Selcon, S. J., & Taylor, R. M. (1990). Evaluation of the situational awareness rating technique (SART) as a tool for aircrew systems design. *AGARD, Situational Awareness in Aerospace Operations, 8, p(SEE N 90-28972 23-53).* AGARD. https://www.sto.nato.int/publications/AGARD/Forms/AGARD%20Document%20Set/docsethomepage.aspx?ID=8332&FolderCTID=0x0120D5200078F9E87043356C409A0D30823AFA16F60B00B8BCE98BB37EB24A8258823D6B11F157&List=03e8ea21-64e6-4d37-8235-04fb61e122e9&RootFolder=%2Fpublications%2FAGARD%2FAGARD%2DCP%2D478

Sirevaag, E., Rohrbaugh, J. W., Stern, J. A., Vedeniapin, A. B., Packingham, K. D., & LaJonchere, C. M. (1999). *Multidimensional characterizations of operator state: A validation of oculomotor metrics (DOT-FAA-AM-99-28).* FAA Office of Aviation Medicine. https://doi.org/10.1037/e412702004-001

Tole, J. R., Stevens, A. T., Harris, R. L., & Ephrath, A. R. (1982). Visual scanning behavior and mental workload in aircraft pilots. *Aviation, Space, and Environmental Medicine, 53*(1), 54–62. PMID: 7055491

Van De Merwe, K., Van Dijk, H., & Zon, R. (2012). Eye movements as an indicator of situation awareness in a flight simulator experiment. *The International Journal of Aviation Psychology, 22*(1), 78–95. https://doi.org/10.1080/10508414.2012.635129

Van Orden, K. F., Jung, T. P., & Makeig, S. (2000). Combined eye activity measures accurately estimate changes in sustained visual task performance. *Biological Psychology, 52*(3), 221–240. https://doi.org/10.1016/S0301-0511(99)00043-5

Van Gerven, P. W., Paas, F., Van Merriënboer, J. J., & Schmidt, H. G. (2004). Memory load and the cognitive pupillary response in aging. *Psychophysiology, 41*(2), 167–174. https://doi.org/10.1111/j.1469-8986.2003.00148.x

Veltman, J. A., & Gaillard, A. W. K. (1998). Physiological workload reactions to increasing levels of task difficulty. *Ergonomics, 41*(5), 656–669. https://doi.org/10.1080/0014 01398186829

Watson, A. B., & Yellott, J. I. (2012). A unified formula for light-adapted pupil size. *Journal of Vision, 12*(10), 12–12. https://doi.org/10.1167/12.10.12

Wickham, H. (2016). *ggplot2: Elegant graphics for data analysis.* Springer. https://doi.org/10.1007/978-3-319-24277-4

Wierwille, W. W., & Eggemeier, F. T. (1993). Recommendations for mental workload measurement in a test and evaluation environment. *Human Factors, 35*(2), 263–281. https://doi.org/10.1177/001872089303500205

Chapter 9
Applications of Cardiac and Electrodermal Activity Assessment in Aviation

Ioana V. Koglbauer and Reinhard Braunstingl

Abstract

The use of psychophysiology has flourished in aviation psychology in the past few decades. Psychophysiological measures of cardiac and electrodermal activation are used in aviation research for assessing operators' state and for a better understanding of the relationship between physiological activation, subjective strain, and performance. An advantage of psychophysiological measures is the possibility to collect them in real time during work without interfering with the task. This chapter describes methods and results of cardiac and electrodermal data collection and analysis in aviation. The sensitivity and reliability of various cardiac and electrodermal parameters in different aviation settings are addressed. Special sections are dedicated to the effects of G-forces during flight and adaptation to microgravity during spaceflight. In addition, applications of cardiac and electrodermal assessment to pilot training and biocybernetics systems (e.g., adaptive automation) are demonstrated. Finally, techniques for data collection and baseline correction are described.

Keywords: psychophysiological assessment, cardiac activity, electrodermal activity, reliability, sensitivity, real flight, spaceflight

Introduction

The measurement of cardiac and electrodermal activity has multiple applications in aviation psychology, ranging from the assessment of performance and training (Kallus & Tropper, 2004; Straussberger et al., 2004; Wilson 2001, 2002), to the design of technical systems, airspace, and procedures (Haarmann et al., 2009; Hilburn & Jorna, 2001; Jorna, 1997; Koglbauer et al., 2014; Parasuraman, 2003; Prinzel et al., 2003). A multilevel approach of psychophysiological assessment including multimodal psychophysiological assessment as well as subjective and performance measures that can provide converging evidence is recommended (Boucsein & Backs, 2009; Hilburn & Jorna, 2001; Kallus & Tropper, 2004; Koglbauer et al., 2011). Parameters of cardiac and electrodermal activity have the advantage of distinguishing between various levels of strain and can be applied in real time without interfering with the task. Psychophysiological measures are objective, because usually they are not under voluntary control and cannot be faked. However, they can be influenced by a series of factors such as the initial state (Kallus, 1992), artifacts (Jorna, 1992), and G-forces (Burton & Whinnery, 1996). Subjective measures of strain can be applied after termination of the task, or during interruptions of the task.

This chapter begins with a presentation of the parameters of cardiac and electrodermal activity, their sensitivity and reliability, and typical applications of cardiac and electrodermal assessment in aviation. Thereafter, two sections address the psychophysiological effects of G-forces on pilots during flight and astronauts' adaptation to microgravity during spaceflight. Special sections are dedicated to applications of cardiac and electrodermal parameters for the assessment of pilot training and for designing adaptive automation. Finally, techniques for cardiac and electrodermal recording and baseline correction are presented.

Applications of Cardiac Activity Assessment in Aviation

The cardiac activity is influenced by the sympathetic and parasympathetic systems. Main parameters of the cardiac activity are: heart rate (HR) measured in beats per minute (bpm), the heart period or inter-beat interval (IBI), measured in milliseconds (ms), and the heart rate variability (HRV). There are different ways of calculating HRV (Jorna, 1992). Formulas include standard deviations, mean square of differences between successive inter-beat intervals, or root of mean square of successive differences. Frequency analysis methods determine HRV from the wave oscillations such as the respiratory sinus arrhythmia and the power of the 0.1-Hz component.

HR is used in psychophysiology as an indicator of physical, mental, and emotional strain (Backs & Boucsein, 2000; De Waard, 1996; Henning & Sauter, 1996; Hidalgo-Muñoz et al., 2018; Jackson & Dishman, 2006; Rousselle et al., 1995; Yasumasu et al., 2006). Several studies have shown that subjective and cardiac measures of workload were comparable (Lee & Liu, 2003). Wilson (2002) found cardiac parameters to be even more sensitive than the subjective measures of workload. In conditions of rest, the reliability of the HRV ($r=.82$) and HR ($r=.91$) is good (Fahrenberg, 2001). A significant HRV reliability coefficient (0.66) was reported also during ergometer exercise (Amara & Wolfe, 1998). In a laboratory study Guijt et al. (2007) reported a good reliability coefficient (0.84) in cycling, acceptable (0.75) in lying down, and excellent (0.94) in the second hour of an ambulatory night rest. Schmidt et al. (2012) reported significant correlations of HRV at rest (0.82) and during speech anticipation (0.85).

The cardiac activity parameters are sensitive to a series of influencing factors such as respiration, muscle activity, body position, physical fitness, and age (Jorna, 1992). These factors need to be considered when selecting participants, specifying data collection procedures and data analysis. A section on techniques at the end of this chapter addresses data collection and analysis that have been successful in aviation settings.

In aviation operations, the cardiac parameters of HR and HRV were shown to be sensitive for distinguishing different levels of strain induced by workload (Boucsein, 2007; Dahlstroem et al., 2011; Hilburn & Jorna, 2001; Jorna, 1997; Lee & Liu, 2003; Magnusson, 2002; Metalis, 1991; Veltman, 2002; Wilson, 2001, 2002). For example, Wilson (2001) recorded the HR of a pilot crew and compared the HR of the pilot in command and his copilot during different flight phases of a real non-commercial flight. Wilson (2001) noted that the pilot in command had a higher HR during landings than the copilot. This was considered an indication of higher workload experienced by the pilot in command as compared with the copilot. Wilson (2001) also observed intra-individual variations during the 1-hr flight: The HR of the pilot in command was 30 bpm higher before landing (high workload) than before the flight (lower workload). During an attempt to land on an iced runway, which was associated with high workload, the mean HR of the pilot in command increased to 150 bpm, being the maximum value measured during the flight. Mean HRs of both pilots increased noticeably in a real emergency during flight. The psychophysiological impact of the flight tasks was stronger in real than in simulated flight (Wilson, 2001), confirming the findings of Jorna (1993).

Dahlstroem et al. (2011) recorded the HR of seven experienced flight instructors during an aerobatic flight. The mean HR of the group of flight instructors was between 95 and 100 bpm during taxi, takeoff, and the first aerobatic session, increasing to 115 bpm during the following aerobatic sequences, and 105 bpm during straight and level flight and decreasing slightly to 100 bpm during the landing (Dahlstroem et al., 2011). The mean HR of the flight instructor group was significantly higher during the aerobatic sequences, which were subjectively rated as being more difficult (Dahlstroem et al., 2011).

Jorna (1997) investigated the "event-related heart rate (EHR)" as an indicator of information processing during discrete pilot tasks where pilots were presented with particular stimuli/events during a simulation. The analysis of the pilots' cardiac activity showed a distinct HR pattern. After the event, pilots' HR decreased shortly during information detection, followed by an increase during information processing and another distinct increase during the response selection and execution.

Kallus and Tropper (2004) examined HR change patterns of 26 male jet pilots during a difficult "black hole approach" from start until 30 s after touchdown in a full-flight simulator. The HR measurement was divided into 13 sections, corresponding to the flight profile. Depending on their landing performance, pilots were assigned to three groups: normal landing, problems, and crash. On average, the pilots' HR was lowest in the group that landed without problems. Pilots that landed with problems had a higher HR as compared with the group without problems. The group of pilots that crashed had the highest HR. Kallus and Tropper (2004) attributed the increased HR to increased strain and stress experienced by the pilots.

Although widely accepted as workload indicators, physiological measures are not considered to measure exclusively workload. Physiological reactivity patterns can be influenced by multiple factors such as different types of work demand and contextual or individual factors (Gaillard et al., 1996). Lackner et al. (2013) reported an increase in HR in participants experiencing positive emotions and amusement. The authors of this chapter observed such a pattern when analyzing real-flight data. Figure 9.1 illustrates the HR of an expert aerobatic pilot during rest before flight and a series of aerobatic maneuvers: loop, hammerhead, Cuban eight, reverse half Cuban, barrel roll, Immelmann, spin, double barrel roll, Dutch rolls, and inverted flight. Although the pilot's HR was higher during flight than during rest, the pilot reported to have experienced low workload and intense joy during the flight. When people experience positive emotion and amusement the HRV is expected to be high. This was also the case of this aerobatic pilot whose HRV was higher during most aerobatic maneuvers than during rest (Figure 9.2). The aerobatic pilot performed pressure breathing and muscle straining to improve his physiological response to G-forces. This example shows that, if used complementarily, the parameters HR and HRV together can give a better indication of the psychophysiological response.

Contrary to HR, the HRV decreases with the increase in mental strain (Boucsein, 2007; Boucsein & Thum, 1996; Hilburn & Jorna, 2001), effort (Schellekens et al., 2000), and task load (Byrne & Parasuraman, 1996). An increase in HRV over time during flight was considered an indication of decreased workload as a result of training (Hidalgo-Muñoz et al., 2018).

In a study with air traffic controllers, Straussberger et al. (2004) reported a decreasing HR and increasing HRV showing a deactivation of air traffic

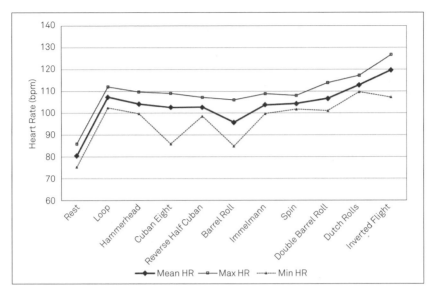

Figure 9.1   HR (bpm) of an aerobatic pilot during rest and during real flight. HR = heart
rate; bpm = beats per minute.

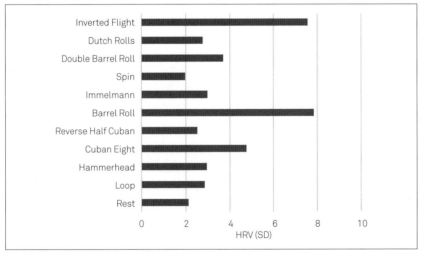

Figure 9.2   HRV (SD) of an aerobatic pilot during rest and during real flight. HRV = heart
rate variability.

controllers in conditions of monotonous traffic repetitiveness and low traffic density. More recently, Mansikka et al. (2016) studied HR and HRV patterns for differentiating between sub-standard performance and high-
performance approaches in fighter pilots. Pilots with high performance in

approaches had a lower HRV than pilots with sub-standard performance (Mansikka et al., 2016).

Applications of Electrodermal Activity Assessment in Aviation

The recording of electrodermal activity (EDA) in real flight emerged in the recent decades. Electrodermal parameters are considered "pure" measures of the sympathetic nervous system (Boucsein, 2012). In laboratory settings, mean skin conductance level (SCL) values of 8.26 μS (SD = 4.64 μS) and an excellent reliability coefficient (0.99) have been reported (Boucsein, 1992). Electrodermal parameters are sensitive to variations of workload during flight (Wilson, 2002). The electrodermal responses (EDR) frequency could differentiate between flight tasks with various workload, but the sum of EDR amplitudes did not show sufficient sensitivity (Wilson, 2002). A high frequency of nonspecific skin conductance reactions (NS.SCR frequency) is an indicator of increased emotional strain (Boucsein, 1991; Boucsein & Backs, 2000) such as anxiety (Boucsein, 2007; Dindo & Fowles, 2008; Flykt et al., 2007; Gavazzeni et al., 2007). NS.SCR frequency rest values between 0 and 10 NS.SCRs/min and activation values of up to 20 NS.SCRs/min have been reported (Boucsein, 1992). Research shows that the short-time reliability of the NS.SCRs frequency is high (r = .81; Fahrenberg & Foerster, 1982). The amplitude of skin conductance reactions (SCR amplitude) is an indicator of mental activity (Boucsein & Backs, 2000; Keil et al., 2008). In addition, SCR amplitude increased in participants watching pleasant and unpleasant pictures as compared with neutral pictures (Bradley et al., 2008). Mean SCR amplitude values of 1.15 μS (SD = 1.02) and a high SCR amplitude reliability (r = .97) were reported in 60 participants during acoustic stimulation in the laboratory (Boucsein, 1992).

Boucsein (2007) analyzed cardiac and electrodermal activation patterns of a pilot during real-flight in a Cessna 172 aircraft. The pilot's increased strain during takeoff and climb was reflected by an increase in SCL, NS.SCR frequency, and SCR amplitude. Another increase in SCL, NS.SCR frequency, and SCR amplitude occurred when the pilot performed steep turns and stalls.

Boucsein and Backs (2009) postulate that psychophysiological parameters of cardiac and electrodermal activity reflect an interplay of four different arousal systems. An increase of HR or NS.SCR frequency and amplitude would show an activation of the affect arousal system (Boucsein & Backs, 2009). A decrease in HRV, or an increase in the recovery time of NS.SCR would be associated with the activation of the effort system that is related to cognitive workload (Boucsein & Backs, 2009). A moderate increase in HR or an increase in NS.SCR amplitude would indicate an activation of the preparatory activation system, thus, increasing readiness for immediate motor actions (Boucsein & Backs, 2009). An accentuated increase in HR, blood pressure, and tonic EDA would indicate an activation of the general arousal system (Boucsein & Backs, 2009). Thus, high, moderate, or low values of physiological parameters can be attributed to the activation of various arousal systems. The interplay of various arousal systems might not be identified with univariate statistical analyses, but may require a qualitative or multivariate approach.

For example, Borghini et al. (2020) have shown that performance, subjective and psychophysiological measures of brain activity, HR, and galvanic skin response – taken individually – were not consistent in differentiating task phases with different workload and stress of air traffic controllers during a realistic simulation (Borghini et al., 2020). Borghini et al. (2020) developed a *fusion-based stress index* using machine learning and merged the psychophysiological parameters. Differences among task phases were significant for the fusion-based stress index.

In summary, research in laboratory, simulator, and real-flight settings shows that cardiac and electrodermal parameters add useful information about the operator's strain induced by work, which is complimentary to subjective and performance measures. However, the physical environment in the aircraft, centrifuge, or spaceflight exposes the human body to additional sources of influence such as G-forces. The following two sections address the effect of G-forces on the physiological parameters.

Acceleration Forces: A Special Issue in Flight Psychophysiology

During flight the human body is exposed to acceleration from different directions (e.g., G-forces). The acceleration force acting on the z-axis (the head-to-feet direction in a standing position) reduces the cerebral blood flow (Burton & Whinnery, 1996). In normal conditions the acceleration on the z-axis is equal to the Earth gravitation force which is $1\,g$ ($9.80665\ m/s^2$). As a consequence of sustained exposure of the human body to forces higher than $4\,g$, loss of peripheral vision ($M=4.10\,g$, $SD=0.70$), black-out or the full loss of vision ($M=4.80\,g$, $SD=0.80$), or loss of consciousness ($M=5.4\,g$, $SD=0.90$) can occur (Burton & Whinnery, 1996). Due to physiological self-regulation, the HR increases during a sustained exposure to more than $2\,g$ in the head-to-feet direction, if no equipment for G-protection is used (Burton & Whinnery, 1996). An increase in HR and a decrease in the inter-beat interval were immediately observed between the first and the second beat after the onset of acceleration (Jauregui-Renaud et al., 2006).

Psychophysiological parameters of HR, HRV (MSSD), and SCL during real flight with variable G-forces were analyzed by the authors of this chapter using data from 29 active male pilots ($M=37.41$, $SD=11.73$ years; Koglbauer, 2009). G-forces on the z-axis were referenced to the pilot in the direction from head to feet. For standardization, physiological recordings from the first 10 s of the recovery phase were analyzed for each maneuver. The acceleration profile of all maneuvers is illustrated in Figure 9.3. Data for rest, flight test, and flight retest values of the parameters HR, HRV (MSSD), and SCL obtained from 29 pilots are presented descriptively in Table 9.1. Significant test–retest correlations of the HR were found for all aircraft recoveries: stall ($r=.74$, $p<.0001$), spin ($r=0.94$, $p<.0001$), upset ($r=.83$, $p<.0001$), and overbanked attitude ($r=.66$, $p<.0001$). In addition, significant test–retest correlations of the HRV (RMMSD) were reported for stall ($\rho=.70$, $p<.0001$), spin ($\rho=.41$, $p<.02$), upset ($\rho=.62$, $p<.0001$), and overbanked attitude ($\rho=.55$, $p<.002$). Test–retest correlations of the mean SCL (µS) were

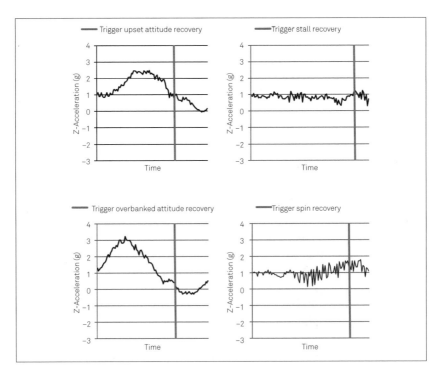

Figure 9.3   Acceleration profile of the flight maneuver. After the start of recovery represented by the vertical trigger line, recovery data are presented for an interval of 10 s.

Table 9.1 Descriptive data of the cardiac and electrodermal activation of pilots (*N* = 29)

Exercise	Test	*M*	*SE*	*Mdn*	95% CI	
					LL	*UL*
Mean HR (bpm)						
Stall	Test	116.37	19.10	116.05	109.10	123.62
	Retest	115.67	16.50	116.08	109.40	121.95
Spin	Test	117.68	20.73	116.77	109.79	125.56
	Retest	113.98	18.01	113.83	107.12	120.82
Unusual attitude	Test	105.63	15.59	104.44	99.70	111.57
	Retest	97.92	16.70	95.58	91.56	104.27
Overbanked attitude	Test	104.13	17.43	102.25	97.50	110.76
	Retest	99.38	15.53	99.05	93.48	105.29
Rest		75.97	9.94	75.70	72.19	79.80
HRV (RMSSD)						
Stall	Test	3.55	3.50	2.50	2.22	4.89
	Retest	3.32	6.00	2.07	1.03	5.60
Spin	Test	3.35	4.00	2.12	1.90	4.90
	Retest	2.24	1.80	1.73	1.60	2.90
Unusual attitude	Test	5.05	4.74	3.09	3.25	6.86
	Retest	6.16	7.32	3.89	3.37	8.95
Overbanked attitude	Test	4.75	4.87	2.93	2.90	6.61
	Retest	6.11	7.48	2.38	3.26	8.96
Rest		6.42	4.23	5.21	4.81	8.03
Mean SCL (µS)						
Stall	Test	14.10	5.76	14.14	11.87	16.26
	Retest	13.64	5.60	13.00	11.50	15.80
Spin	Test	13.92	5.81	14.48	11.71	16.13
	Retest	13.52	5.52	12.90	11.42	15.62
Unusual attitude	Test	14.40	6.04	13.48	12.10	16.70
	Retest	14.97	6.79	15.08	12.39	17.55
Overbanked attitude	Test	14.12	5.81	13.06	11.91	16.33
	Retest	13.83	5.73	13.09	11.65	16.01
Rest		11.14	3.92	10.52	9.65	12.63

Note. bpm = beats per minute; CI = confidence interval; HR = heart rate; HRV = heart rate variability; *LL* = lower limit; RRMSD = root mean square of successive R-R interval differences; *UL* = upper limit; SCL = skin conductance level.

also significant for aircraft recovery from stall (r=.98, p<.0001), spin (r=0.94, p<.0001), upset (r=.93, p<.0001), and overbanked attitude (r=.99, p<.0001). These results demonstrate the test–retest reliability of HR, HRV (root mean square of successive R-R interval differences [RMSSD]), and SCL for flight with variable G-forces.

Acceleration and Adaptation to Spaceflight

During spaceflight, astronauts experience considerably different environmental conditions such as G-forces (microgravity), radiation, altered lighting, and light–dark cycles (Kanas & Manzey, 2008). The human cardiovascular system is adapted to the gravity on Earth. According to Kanas and Manzey (2008):

- In humans, a hydrostatic pressure gradient develops along the vertical body axis, with the arterial blood pressure increasing from head (about 70 mmHg) to feet (about 200 mmHg). Both the heart and blood vessels work against this effect of gravity. (p. 17).
- As a physiological adaptation to microgravity experienced in space, the pump activity of the heart decreases.

The HR of three astronauts was recorded in 48-hr intervals in three phases: before launch, during spaceflight, and after landing (Liu et al., 2015). As illustrated in Figure 9.4, the astronauts' maximum HR decreased during spaceflight and increased after the flight (Liu et al., 2015). The decrease in maximum HR during spaceflight was associated with a decrease in body trunk activity and rhythmicity (Liu et al., 2015).

Baevsky et al. (2011) assessed the HRV during long space missions on the International Space Station (ISS) of 14 male astronauts aged between 35 and 54 years. The astronauts' HRV was relatively stable during 6 months in space, but an impairment of HRV was reported toward the end of the spaceflight. This, according to the authors, may impair the re-adaptation of the astronauts after landing on Earth.

Astronauts' HR and HRV were mainly assessed as an indicator of physiological self-regulation during spaceflight. However, astronauts are exposed to a series of positive and negative psychological stressors (Blackwell Landon et al., 2017; Kanas & Manzey, 2008) and the strain experienced can be also reflected in the astronauts' cardiac activity. Early in 1969 NASA recorded and reported the HR of the astronauts during the entire Apollo 11 spaceflight, the first lunar landing mission. The HR data were reported for various phases of the mission. The commander's mean HR was 71 bpm during the entire mission and 110 bpm during the entire lunar surface exploration (NASA, 1969). A peak of 160 bpm in the commander's HR was recorded at

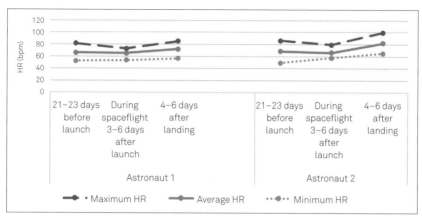

Figure 9.4   Effect of spaceflight on astronaut's HR. HR = heart rate; bpm = beats per minute. Data from Liu et al., 2015.

the termination of the first activity on the moon. The commander's HR values ranged between 68 and 120 bpm during ascent and between 100 and 150 bpm during descent (NASA, 1969).

Psychophysiological Assessment of Training Effects

For the evaluation of an anticipation-based flight training program, Koglbauer et al. (2011) collected psychophysiological, subjective, and performance data in a multilevel approach. The anticipation-based method is described in Chapter 4 by Koglbauer and Braunstingl (2021) in this volume. Three EDA parameters – SCL, NS.SCR frequency, mean SCR amplitude – and two cardiac parameters – HR (bpm) and HRV (MSSD) – were collected from 33 pilots during simulated and real flight. They used a pretest–training–posttest design with an experimental and a control group. Subjective workload was self-assessed by pilots using the NASA Task Load Index (Hart & Staveland, 1988) and emotion was self-assessed using the Positive and Negative Affect Schedule (Watson & Clark, 1988). Performance measures were instructor ratings and task completion time. The results give a comprehensive picture of the positive training effects. Pilots from the experimental group performed the maneuvers better and faster than pilots from the control group. In the posttest, pilots from the experimental group showed higher HRV and reported lower workload than pilots from the control group (Koglbauer et al., 2011). Workload and HR decreased in both groups after repeated test sessions. This is also confirmed by Hidalgo-Muñoz et al. (2018), who reported a decrease in HR with time on task as a training effect. Koglbauer et al. (2011) reported that pilots' HR during flight tests was significantly higher in the aircraft as compared with the fixed-base simulator. This effect was attributed to higher physical demand and G-forces experienced in the aircraft. Higher SCR amplitude was observed in the experimental group, indicating higher preparatory activation (Boucsein & Backs, 2009) as a result of the anticipation-based training concept. On average, pilots from the experimental group had a lower NS.SCR frequency than pilots from the control group, indicating lower affect arousal as a psychophysiological training effect. Individuals with a lower NS.SCR frequency are less prone to attention tunneling and stress-related behavioral inhibition responses (Boucsein & Backs, 2009). SCL, considered an indicator of general arousal, increased with practice during tests in both groups. Higher SCL was associated with better engagement and performance (Koglbauer et al., 2011). An increased SCL was also reported in drivers who successfully avoided obstacles than in drivers who crashed in a critical situation (Collet et al., 2005). Pilots' positive emotions such as excitement, feeling of strength, pride, and enthusiasm were stronger after repeated flight tests. Thus, the use of psychophysiological measures in a multilevel approach gives a better understanding of training effects than do performance and subjective measures.

Another application is described by Mansikka et al. (2016), who proposed the use of pilots' HR and HRV in addition to performance evaluations as part of the proficiency tests of Air Force pilots. Physiological measures of HR and HRV were considered to improve the examiner's awareness of pilots' ability and spare capacity to manage higher workload. In a study with 26 volunteer male Air Force F/A-18 pilots, Mansikka et al. (2016) demonstrated that variations in pilots' HR and HRV could identify pilots who, despite good performance, experienced greater strain induced by mission segments with high workload. Increased workload is associated with a decrease in spare mental capacity that pilots may need to cope with additional or unexpected task demands.

Thus, these examples show that psychophysiological measures can be used by training organizations for calibrating an optimal and cost-effective training duration. Pilots who demonstrate proficiency and high strain during exercises can benefit from additional exercises. Pilots who demonstrate proficiency and low strain may be ready to start practicing at a higher level of difficulty or move to a new skill.

Adaptive Automation: A Special Application of Psychophysiology in Aviation

As the measures of cardiac and electrodermal activity have been sensitive to evaluate pilots' workload, researchers have attempted to use these data in real time as an input to the technical system in aviation (Haarmann et al., 2009; Parasuraman, 2003; Prinzel et al., 2003) and other domains (Dijksterhuis et al., 2012). In *adaptive automation*, different values of cardiac and electrodermal activation are used as triggers for adjusting the amount of automation support. The scope is to achieve an optimal level of workload and keep the operator in the loop, in control of the situation. The biocybernetic adaptive system can increase the level of automation and decrease the task load when the psychophysiological trigger indicates excessive workload in the human operators (e.g., pilots). In turn, the biocybernetic adaptive system can reduce the level of automation and increase the need for manual control when the psychophysiological trigger indicates that workload is too low.

The method is described using the example of a simple biocybernetic adaptive system in an IFR flight simulator (Haarmann et al., 2009). For each individual operator a physiological range with upper and lower thresholds of the parameters EDR freq, HR, and HRV was calculated and used to trigger the adaptive automation. For each parameter, Haarmann et al. (2009) used four physiological recordings with a length of 2 min: two low-workload periods (IFR flight without turbulences) and two high-workload periods (IFR flight with maximal turbulences). The individual upper and lower thresholds were calculated as the arithmetic mean of the recording periods. During flight, physiological data were recorded and the physiological parameters were calculated in real time every 2 min. Adaptive automation was performed when the actual 2-min average values of the physiological parameters were below and above the individual set point. The level of turbulence was manipulated to induce workload variations.

Haarmann et al. (2009) tested three combinations of psychophysiological parameters for initiating adaptive automation: *EDR frequency alone*, *EDR frequency AND HR*, and *EDR frequency AND HRV*. The most efficient combination was EDR frequency AND HRV (Haarmann et al., 2009).

Techniques for Collection and Analysis of Cardiac and Electrodermal Activity

Techniques of Physiological Recording

In applied settings the techniques of physiological data recording may require tests and adjustments, depending on the objective and conditions of assessment. For example, Koglbauer (2009) recorded pilots' electrocardiogram (ECG) and EDA during simulated and real flight using the Varioport system (Becker Meditec, Karlsruhe, Germany). A trigger was set manually by the flight instructor and recoded with the physiological data, thus, allowing different phases of the flight task to be identified in the physiological recording. In addition, an on-board video of the flight was recorded and used as a back-up for datasets where a trigger may be missing or further clarification may be needed.

Recording of Cardiac Activity

Koglbauer (2009) recorded pilots' ECG during real flight with high G-forces. After a series of tests, a bi-axillar thorax lead was used for the ECG, to avoid artifacts induced by pressure on the electrodes from belts of the emergency parachute (Figure 9.5a) and seat harnesses (Figure 9.5b). The

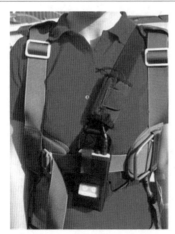 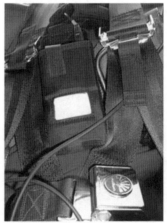

a. On the ground with the emergency parachute and the Varioport device

b. In the aerobatic aircraft with emergency parachute and fastened harnesses

Figure 9.5   Verification and documentation of potential disturbances on physiological measurement during real flight tests. The electrodes need to be free of mechanical disturbances such as those potentially induced by harnesses.

thorax lead used a sampling frequency of 512 Hz and a saving frequency of 256 Hz.

However, the ECG electrodes may not be affected in simulator or in an aircraft with another type of harness. Veltman (2002), for example, recorded pilots' ECG using two Ag/AgCl electrodes, one attached under the heart and one attached at the right collar bone.

Recording of Electrodermal Activity

EDA is normally recorded from palmar or plantar skin (Boucsein, 1992). If both hands are used by the participants for performing tasks during the trials and pressure on the electrodes is expected, the recording from plantar skin is recommendable. Koglbauer (2009) recorded pilots' EDA during real flight from the plantar sites of the left foot as described by Boucsein (1992; Fig. 28). Two Ag/Ag-Cl-electrodes with 22-mm diameter (1 cm^2 measurement area) were used. The electrodes were filled with 0.5 % NaCl paste and allowed to stabilize for 10 min before being attached to the skin. Recording was performed with 0.5-V constant voltage and with a resolution of 0.002 µS. The EDA signal was stored with a sampling frequency of 512 Hz, but the saving frequency was reduced to 64 Hz. The SCL (µS) was processed with the software EDA-Vario, Version 1.8 (Schaefer, 2007).

Baseline Correction of Physiological Data

When different groups of participants are compared, the interindividual differences can be a source of variance that confounds the variance induced by the test conditions. In such conditions the calculation of an initial or baseline measurement for correction of the physiological data is required. For example, the mean over all the recorded test values can be used as a *baseline* value. Alternatively, multiple rest measurements can be used to calculate a baseline. Koglbauer et al. (2011) collected several rest measurements of 2 min from pilots participating in an experiment before and after each flight simulator session. During the rest measurements the participants were told to relax, sit quietly on a chair, with their eyes closed. Data from rest measurements (e.g., before test, between tests, and after the tests) were used to calculate mean and standard deviation (SD) values for each individual participant.

Baseline scores can be biased by the initial state of the participants (Kallus, 1992; see also Chapter 6 on reactivity by Uhlig and Uhlig in this volume) and anticipative processes related to the experiment and the rest measurement itself. In practice, the first rest measurement often shows higher arousal than the subsequent measurements and is excluded from calculating the correction. Several rest measurements collected after the experiment or test may be best because these may be associated with feelings of relief, relaxation, habituation etc. However, depending on the length and intensity of the test, the posttest rest measurements could be also associated with fatigue.

The procedure for baseline correction depends on the data and there is no generally applicable rule for calculating it (Fahrenberg et al., 1979). An example for the calculation of the baseline correction is given by Koglbauer et al. (2011). The following formula exemplifies the procedure for HR:

$$V = (HR_t - M_b)/SD_b$$

where V is the baseline corrected value of an individual participant, HR_t is the absolute mean test value of the individual participant, M_b is the mean value of the baseline measurements of the individual participant, and SD_b is the standard deviation of the baseline measurements of the individual participant.

Using this or other formulas, test data from each individual can be corrected and used for comparisons between groups of individuals.

Instructions and Ethical Considerations

The experimenter can use instructions before a participant's attendance to avoid confounding influences on the participant's physiological activity. Before the experiment participants should be instructed to obtain sufficient sleep, not to drink coffee or energy drinks, not to take medication and to report any medication taken. Before aerobatic flight, participants should be instructed to consume a light and small meal. Instructions and experimental procedures need to be tried out to ensure that they are understandable. Participants should also be instructed to inform the experimenter if anything unusual happened during the experiment or during a break. In addition, the experimenter should make a plausibility check of the physiological data and try to identify the reason for unusual peaks (e.g., falling objects, startling noises, or running to renew a parking ticket).

Knowledge and acceptance of physiological measures, especially of the ECG, have improved in recent years. Many participants in experiments use heart monitors for fitness, know their rest HR values and the HR values of their fitness training zone. However, pilots and air traffic controllers are subject to recurrent medical examinations required in addition to proficiency checks and may be worried about possible negative consequences of an experimental measurement. Thus, aviation psychologists should consider explaining to pilots and controllers that their physiological data will not be used for medical assessment purposes, and medical doctors or supervisors will not have access to these data. Psychophysiological data files should be de-identified: No names, only codes should be used. When data are collected for an approved training organization, performance data must be collected with names, according to their standard procedures. However, subjective and psychophysiological data can be collected anonymously, using codes. Experimental data should be analyzed and presented for the group, and not for the individual. If the participants want, they should be able to receive a copy of the analyzed group data. Informed consent should be obtained from the participants, according to international ethical guidelines. In addition, most research organizations have an ethical and data protection committee that verifies the experimental procedures. Last, but not least, it is important to inform participants about the subject of investigation. Especially, if the experiment is not testing the skills or competence of the participants, but the effect of a training program, new equipment, or a new airspace design. For example, a licensed aviation operator self-rated their workload as 0 in every test, being afraid that a higher workload would make them look less competent. However, the experimenter would have interpreted higher workload as an indicator of poor system design. Although measurements of performance, subjective strain, and physiological activity are collected, they are dependent on the experimental variables (e.g., training methods, equipment or environmental conditions).

Conclusion

This chapter presented methods and techniques of cardiac and electrodermal assessment in aviation psychophysiology. Typical applications of psychophysiology are in the assessment of task load, training effects, and system design in a multilevel approach, complimentary to subjective and performance measures. As research shows, the parameters of cardiac and electrodermal activity are sensitive to various levels of mental, physical, and emotional strain and can be reliably collected in special aviation settings (e.g., real flight with variable G-forces). However, the methods applied need to eliminate or control for possible artifacts (Jorna, 1992), and special techniques for data recording and baseline correction may be required. Future trends are the application of psychophysiological measures in biocybernetics systems and in the calibration of optimal and cost-effective training duration.

References

Amara, C. E., & Wolfe, L. A. (1998). Reliability of noninvasive methods to measure cardiac autonomic function. *Canadian Journal of Applied Physiology, 23*(4), 396–408. https://doi.org/10.1139/h98-024

Backs, R. W., & Boucsein, W. (2000). *Engineering psychophysiology. Issues and applications.* Lawrence Erlbaum. https://doi.org/10.1201/b12463

Baevsky, R. M., Chernikova, A. G., Funtova, I. I., & Tank, J. (2011). Assessment of individual adaptation to microgravity during long term space flight based on stepwise discriminant analysis of heart rate variability parameters. *Acta Astronautica, 69*(11–12), 1148–1152. https://doi.org/10.1016/j.actaastro.2011.07.011

Blackwell Landon, L., Rokholt, C., Slack, K. J., & Pecena, Y. (2017). Selecting astronauts for long-duration exploration missions: Considerations for team performance and functioning. *REACH – Reviews in Human Space Exploration, 5*, 33–56. https://doi.org/10.1016/j.reach.2017.03.002

Borghini, G., Di Flumeri, G., Aricò, P., Sciaraffa, N., Bonelli, S., Ragosta, M., Tomasello, P., Drogoul, F., Turhan, U., Acikel, B., Ozan, A., Imbert, J. P., Granger, G., Benhacene, R., & Babiloni, F. (2020). A multimodal and signals fusion approach for assessing the impact of stressful events on air traffic controllers. *Nature, 8600*(10), 1–18. https://doi.org/10.1038/s41598-020-65610-z

Boucsein, W. (1991). Electrodermal activity as an indicator in the psychopharmacological treatment of anxiety: theoretical background and empirical results. *Pharmacopsychoecologia, 4* (1-2), 23–32.

Boucsein, W. (1992). *Electrodermal activity.* Plenum Press. https://doi.org/10.1007/978-1-4757-5093-5

Boucsein, W. (2012). *Electrodermal activity* (2nd ed.). Springer. https://doi.org/10.1007/978-1-4614-1126-0

Boucsein, W. (2007). Psychphysiologie im Flug – eine Fallstudie [Flight psychophysiology – A case study]. In P. G. Richter, R. Rau, & S. Mühlpfordt (Eds.), *Arbeit und Gesundheit. Zum aktuellen Stand in einem Forschungs- und Praxisfeld* [Work and Health. Current Research and Practice] (pp. 130–144). Pabst Science.

Boucsein, W., & Backs, R. W. (2000). Engineering psychophysiology as a discipline: Historical and theoretical aspects. In R. W. Backs, & W. Boucsein (Eds.), *Engineering Psychophysiology. Issues and Applications* (pp. 3–30). Lawrence Erlbaum. https://doi.org/10.1201/b12463

Boucsein, W., & Backs, W. (2009). The psychophysiology of emotion, arousal, and personality: methods and models. In V. G. Duffy (Ed.) *Handbook of digital human modeling. Research for applied ergonomics and human factors engineering* (pp. 35-1/35-8). CRC Press, Taylor & Francis.

Boucsein, W., & Thum, M. (1996). Multivariate psychophysiological analysis of stress-strain processes during different break schedules during computer work. In J. Fahrenberg, & M. Myrtek (Eds.), *Ambulatory assessment* (pp. 305–313). Hogrefe & Huber.

Bradley, M. M., Miccoli, L., Escrig, M., & Lang, P. (2008). The pupil as a measure of emotional arousal and autonomic activation. *Psychophysiology, 45*(2), 602–607. https://doi.org/10.1111/j.1469-8986.2008.00654.x

Burton, R. R., & Whinnery, J. E. (1996). Biodynamics: Sustained acceleration. In R. L. De Hart (Ed.), *Fundamentals of aerospace medicine* (2nd ed., pp. 202–249). Williams & Wilkins.

Byrne, E. A., & Parasuraman, R. (1996). Psychophysiology and adaptive automation. *Biological Psychology, 42*(3), 249–268. https://doi.org/10.1016/0301-0511(95)05161-9

Collet, C., Petit, C., Priez, A., & Dittmar, A. (2005). Stroop color-word test, arousal, electrodermal activity and performance in a critical driving situation. *Biological Psychology, 69*(2), 195–203. https://doi.org/10.1016/j.biopsycho.2004.07.003

Dahlstroem, N., Naehlinder, S., Wilson, G. F., & Svensson, E. (2011). Recording of psychophysiological data during aerobatic training. *International Journal of Aviation Psychology, 21*(2), 105–122. https://doi.org/10.1080/10508414.2011.556443

De Waard, D. (1996). *The measurement of drivers' mental workload*. The Traffic Research Centre VSC, University of Groningen.

Dijksterhuis, C., Stuiver, A., Mulder, B., Brookhuis, K. A., & de Waard, D. (2012). An adaptive driver support system: User experiences and driving performance in a simulator. *Human Factors, 54*(5), 772–785. https://doi.org/10.1177%2F0018720811430502

Dindo, L., & Fowles, D. C. (2008). The skin conductance orienting response to semantic stimuli: significance can be independent of arousal. *Psychophysiology, 45*(1), 111–118. https://doi.org/10.1111/j.1469-8986.2007.00604.x

Fahrenberg, J., & Foerster, F. (1982). Covariation and consistency of activation parameters. *Biological Psychology, 15*(3–4), 151–169. https://doi.org/10.1016/0301-0511(82)90039-4

Fahrenberg, J., Walschburger, P., Foerster, F., Myrtek, M., & Mueller, W. (1979). *Psychophysiologische Aktivierungsforschung. Ein Beitrag zu den Grundlagen der multivariaten Emotions- und Stress-Theorie* [Psychophysiological activation research. A contribution to the basics of multivariate emotion and stress theory]. Minerva.

Fahrenberg, J. (2001). Grundlagen und Methoden der Psychophysiologie [Fundamentals and methods of psychophysiology]. In F. Rössler (Ed.), *Enzyklopädie der Psychologie* (Vol. 4, pp. 317–483). Hogrefe.

Flykt, A., Esteves, F., & Öhman, A. (2007). Skin conductance responses to masked conditioned stimuli: phylogenetic/ontogenetic factors versus direction of threat? *Biological Psychology, 74*(3), 328–336. https://doi.org/10.1016/j.biopsycho.2006.08.004

Gaillard, A. W. K., Boucsein, W., & Stern, J. (1996). Psychophysiology of workload. *Biological Psychology, 42*(3), 245–247. https://doi.org/10.1016/S0301-0511(96)90003-4

Gavazzeni, J., Wiens, S., & Fischer, H. (2007). Age effects to negative arousal differ for self-report and electrodermal activity. *Psychophysiology, 45*(1), 148–151. https://doi.org/10.1111/j.1469-8986.2007.00596.x

Guijt, A. M., Sluiter, J. K., & Frings-Dresen, M. H. W. (2007). Test-retest reliability of heart rate variability and respiration rate at rest and during light physical activity in normal subjects. *Archives of Medical Research, 38*(1), 113–120. https://doi.org/10.1016/j.arcmed.2006.07.009

Haarmann, A., Boucsein, W., & Schaefer, F. (2009). Combining electrodermal responses and cardiovascular measures for probing adaptive automation during simulated flight. *Applied Ergonomics, 40*(6), 1026–1040. https://doi.org/10.1016/j.apergo.2009.04.011

Hart, S. G., & Staveland, L. E. (1988). Development of NASA-TLX (Task Load Index): Results of empirical and theoretical research. In P. A. Hancock & N. Meshkati (Eds.),

Human mental workload (pp. 239–250). North Holland Press. https://doi.org/10.1016/S0166-4115(08)62386-9

Henning, R. A., & Sauter, S. L. (1996). Work-physiological synchronization as a determinant of performance in repetitive computer work. *Biological Psychology, 42*(3), 269–286. https://doi.org/10.1016/0301-0511(95)05162-7

Hidalgo-Muñoz, A. R., Mouratille, D., Matton, N., Causse, M., Rouillard, Y., El-Yagoubi, R. (2018). Cardiovascular correlates of emotional state, cognitive workload and time on-task effect during a realistic flight simulation. *International Journal of Psychophysiology, 128*, 62–69. https://doi.org/10.1016/j.ijpsycho.2018.04.002

Hilburn, B., & Jorna, P. (2001). Workload and air traffic control. In P. A. Hancock & P. A. Desmond (Eds.), *Stress, workload and fatigue: Theory, research and practice* (pp. 384–394). Lawrence Erlbaum Associates.

Jackson, E. M., & Dishman, R. K. (2006). Cardiorespiratory fitness and laboratory stress: a meta-regression analysis. *Psychophysiology, 43*(1), 57–72. https://doi.org/10.1111/j.1469-8986.2006.00373.x

Jauregui-Renaud, K., Reynolds, R., Bronstein, A. M., & Gresty, M. A. (2006). Cardio-respiratory responses evoked by transient linear acceleration. *Aviation, Space and Environmental Medicine, 77*(2), 114–120.

Jorna, P. G. A. M. (1997). *Pilot performance in automated cockpits: Demonstration of event-related heart rate responses to data link applications.* NLR-TP-97639 U. NLR.

Jorna, P. G. A. M. (1992). Spectral analysis of heart rate and psychological state: A review of its validity as a workload index. *Biological Psychology, 34*(2–3), 237–257. https://doi.org/10.1016/0301-0511(92)90017-O

Jorna, P. G. A. M. (1993). Heart rate and workload variations in actual and simulated flight. *Ergonomics, 36*, 1043–1054. https://doi.org/10.1080/00140139308967976

Kallus, K. W. (1992). *Beanspruchung und Ausgangszustand* [The strain and the initial value]. Psychologie Verlags-Union.

Kallus, K. W., & Tropper, K. (2004). Evaluation of a spatial disorientation simulator training for jet pilots. *International Journal of Applied Aviation Studies, 4*(1), 45–55.

Kanas, N., & Manzey, D. (2008). *Space psychology and psychiatry.* Springer. https://doi.org/10.1007/978-1-4020-6770-9

Keil, A., Smith, J. C., Wangelin, B. C., Sabatinelli, D., Bradley, M. M., & Lang, P. (2008). Electrocortical and electrodermal responses covary as a function of motional arousal: a single-trial analysis. *Psychophysiology, 45*(4), 516–523. https://doi.org/10.1111/j.1469-8986.2008.00667.x

Koglbauer, I. (2009). *Multidimensional approach of threat and error management training for VFR pilots.* Doctoral Dissertation. University of Graz, Austria.

Koglbauer, I., Braunstingl, R., Fruehwirth, K., Grubmueller, E., & Loesch, S. (2014). Gender issues in usability of glass cockpit for General Aviation aircraft. In D. Bridges, J. Neal-Smith, & A. J. Mills (Eds.), *Absent aviators: Gender issues in aviation* (pp. 239–260). Ashgate Publishing.

Koglbauer, I., Kallus, K. W., Braunstingl, R., & Boucsein, W. (2011). Recovery training in simulator improves performance and psychophysiological state of pilots during simulated and real visual flight rules flight. *International Journal of Aviation Psychology, 21*(4), 307–324. https://doi.org/10.1080/10508414.2011.606741

Koglbauer, I. V., & Braunstingl, R. (2021). Anticipation-Based Methods for Pilot Training and Aviation Systems Engineering. In I. V. Koglbauer, & S. Biede-Straussberger (Eds.), *Aviation Psychology: Applied Methods and Techniques* (pp. 51–67). Hogrefe.

Lackner, H. K., Weiss, E. M., Schulter, G., Hinghofer-Szalkay, H., Samson, A., Papousek, I. (2013). I got it! Transient cardiovascular response to the perception of humor. *Biological Psychology, 93*(1), 33–40. https://doi.org/10.1016/j.biopsycho.2013.01. 014

Lee, Y. H., & Liu, B. S. (2003). Inflight workload assessment: Comparison of subjective and physiological measurements. *Aviation, Space and Environmental Medicine, 74*(10), 1078–1084.

Liu, Z., Wan, Y., Zhang, L., Tian, Y., Lv, K., Li, Y., Wang, C., Chen, X., Chen, S., & Guo, J. (2015). Alterations in the heart rate and activity rhythms of three orbital astronauts on a space mission. *Life Sciences in Space Research, 4*, 62–66. https://doi.org/10.1016/j. lssr.2015.01.001

Magnusson, S. (2002). Similarities and differences in psychophysiological reactions between simulated and real air-to-ground missions. *International Journal of Aviation Psychology, 12*(1), 49–61. https://doi.org/10.1207/S15327108IJAP1201_5

Mansikka, H., Virtanen, K., Harris, D., & Simola, P. (2016). Fighter pilots' heart rate, heart rate variation and performance during an instrument flight rules proficiency test. *Applied Ergonomics, 56*, 213–219. https://doi.org/10.1016/j.apergo.2016.04.006

Metalis, S. A. (1991). Heart period as a useful index of pilot workload in commercial transport aircraft. *International Journal of Aviation Psychology, 1*(2), 107–116. https://doi. org/10.1207/s15327108ijap0102_2

NASA. (1969). *Apollo 11 mission report.* Manned Spacecraft Center. https://www.hq.nasa. gov/alsj/a11/A11_PAOMissionReport.html

Parasuraman, R. (2003). Adaptive automation matched to human mental workload. In G. R. J. Hockey, A. W. K. Gaillard, & O. Burov (Eds.), *Operator functional state* (pp. 177–193). IOS Press.

Prinzel, L. J., III, Parasuraman, R., Freeman, F. G., Scerbo, M. W., Mikulka, P. J., & Pope, A. T. (2003). *Three experiments examining the use of electroencephalogram, event related potentials, and heart-rate variability for real-time human-centered adaptive automation design. NASA/TP-2003-212442.* NASA Langley Research Center.

Rousselle, J. G., Blascovic, J., & Kelsey, R. M. (1995). Cardiorespiratory response under combined psychological and exercise stress. *International Journal of Psychophysiology, 20*(1), 49–58. https://doi.org/10.1016/0167-8760(95)00026-O

Schaefer, F. (2007). *Software Program EDA-Vario, Version 1.8.* University of Wuppertal, Germany.

Schellekens, J. M. H., Sijtsma, G. J., Vegter, E., & Meijman, T. F. (2000). Immediate and delayed after-effects of long lasting mentally demanding work. *Biological Psychology, 53*(1), 37–56. https://doi.org/10.1016/S0301-0511(00)00039-9

Schmidt, L. A., Santesso, D. L., Miskovic, V., Methewson, K. J., McCabe, R. E., Antony, M. M., & Moscovitch, D. A. (2012). Test-retest reliability of regional electroencephalogram (EEG) and cardiovascular measures in social anxiety disorder (SAD). *International Journal of Psychophysiology, 84*(1), 65–73. https://doi.org/10.1016/j.ijpsycho.2012. 01.011

Straussberger, S., Schaefer, D., & Kallus, K. W. (2004). A psychophysiological investigation of the concept of monotony in ATC: Effects of traffic repetitiveness and traffic density. In ICRAT (Ed.), *Proceedings of 1st International Conference on Research in Air Transportation (ICRAT)* (pp. 199–208). University of Zilina.

Veltman, J. A. (2002). A comparative study of psychophysiological reactions during simulator and real flight. *International Journal of Aviation Psychology, 12*(1), 33–48. https://doi.org/10.1207/S15327108IJAP1201_4

Watson, D., & Clark, L. A. (1988). Development and validation of brief measures of positive and negative affect: The PANAS Scales. *Journal of Personality and Social Psychology, 54*(6), 1063–1070. https://doi.org/10.1037/0022-3514.54.6.1063

Wilson, G. F. (2001). In-flight psychophysiological monitoring. In J. Fahrenberg, & M. Myrthek (Eds.), *Progress in ambulatory assessment* (pp. 435–454). Hogrefe & Huber.

Wilson, G. F. (2002). An analysis of mental workload in pilots during flight using multiple psychophysiological measures. *International Journal of Aviation Psychology, 12*(1), 3–18. https://doi.org/10.1207/S15327108IJAP1201_2

Yasumasu, T., Reyes del Paso, G. A., Takahara, K., & Nakashima, Y. (2006). Reduced baroreflex cardiac sensitivity predicts increased cognitive performance. *Psychophysiology, 43*(1), 41–45. https://doi.org/10.1111/j.1469-8986.2006.00377.x

Contributors

Editors

Ioana V. Koglbauer received her PhD in psychology in 2009 and a habilitation in psychology in 2018 both from the University of Graz, Austria. She is also an experienced aviation psychologist accredited by the European Association for Aviation Psychology (EAAP). Ioana worked several years in teaching and research at Graz University of Technology in Austria, and was a visiting professor at the Institut Supérieur de l'Aéronautique et de l'Espace (ISAE-SUPAERO) in Toulouse, France. She is a passionate experienced in teaching human performance and safety for the Airline Transport Pilot License (ATPL) and Type Rating Instructor (TRI) courses. Ioana has led multiple research projects between academia and the aviation industry, and has authored numerous publications on various topics of aviation psychology and human factors. She was Editor-in-Chief of the peer-reviewed journal *Aviation Psychology and Applied Human Factors* and a member of the Board of the Directors of the European Association for Aviation Psychology (EAAP) for 4 years (2014–2018). In addition, Ioana serves as an expert for various international organizations: the Civil Air Navigation Services Organization (CANSO) and the Human Factors Collaborative Analysis Group of the European Union Aviation Safety Agency (EASA HF CAG). She is currently affiliated with the Air Navigation Service Provider of the Irish Aviation Authority in Dublin, Ireland.

Sonja Biede-Straussberger is Expert for Cognitive Psychology in the Human Factors & Ergonomics department of Airbus Operations. She received her PhD in psychology in 2006, and holds a master's degree in educational science, both from the Karl Franzens University of Graz, Austria. Between 2003 and 2006, her studies with EUROCONTROL were focused on the identification of contributing factors to monotony in air traffic controllers. She then extended her views to the global aeronautical system, when looking at questions of authorities and responsibilities for new aviation concepts together in a French multidisciplinary and cross-industry project. Between 2009 and 2018 she led the Airbus human factors contribution to SESAR, with the endeavor to give human operators a central role throughout the engineering cycle, by taking the complete dimension of psychology into account. Beyond that, she is actively involved in promoting human factors integration in the aviation industry, such as the French Association for System Engineering and regular publications. In the past, she was officer of the Human Factors and Ergonomics Society Europe Chapter, and is currently active to support the European Association for Aviation Psychology

(EAAP). She holds a private pilot license and taught human factors for student pilots as well as courses to engineers. Today, she applies her expertise to continuously improving or developing new products by optimizing the contribution of human factors along all phases of cockpit design.

Authors

Thierry Baccino is a full professor of cognitive psychology in digital technologies at the University of Paris VIII and scientific director of LUTIN (EA 4004) located at the National Museum of Sciences and Techniques in Paris. Thierry Baccino obtained his PhD in cognitive psychology from the University of Aix-en-Provence in 1991 with grants from the National IBM Research Centre. Afterwards he moved as a research assistant to the University of Dundee to study the cognitive processes involved in digital reading. He became assistant professor at the University of Nice Sophia-Antipolis (UNS) in 1993 and full professor in 1998. At the UNS, he founded the Laboratory of Experimental Psychology in 1995 and managed it until 2002. After several visiting professorships (Pavia, Dortmund, Turin, Valencia), he received a Fulbright award in 2004 to work at the Institute for Cognitive Science (University of Colorado at Boulder, USA). He received a CNRS delegation in 2009 and he is currently vice-chair at the European DG Research and at different French research institutes (ANR, HCERES). His research focus is mainly on reading processes using the eye-tracking technique that is often combined with other physiological techniques (EEG, RED, ECG, MOCAP, etc.).

Cedric Bach is a senior human factors specialist at HDG (Human Design Group), a French consulting agency in ergonomics and human factors. He completed his PhD in cognitive ergonomics at the French Institute in Computer Sciences and Control in Paris (2004). For 16 years, his academic research topics deal with usability engineering in different domains such as aeronautics, space, mobile technologies, virtual environments, and complex interactive systems. As a human factors specialist, he analyzes on a daily basis models and designs and evaluates different types of human–systems integrations especially in the aeronautics field and recently for the nuclear industry.

Reinhard Braunstingl received a PhD degree in mechanical engineering from Graz University of Technology, Austria, in 1991. He is a professor at the Graz University of Technology, specialized in mechanics, flight mechanics, and flight simulation. In 2008, Reinhard Braunstingl established the research platform Flight Simulation at Graz University of Technology where he conducted numerous research projects in cooperation with the aviation industry. Reinhard is a visiting professor at the Universidad de Huelva in Spain. He is also an experienced and passioned pilot, flight instructor, and flight examiner. He was the Austrian aerobatics champion in 2009 in the Sportsman Category.

Marie-Christine Bressolle graduated with a PhD in ergonomics from the University of Toulouse 2 in 2000, with a specific interest in cognitive ergonomics and a master's degree in psychology. Working in the field of air traffic control for around 12 years, in the framework of introducing new decision aids, her thesis was related to the building of a shared cognitive environment by en-route air traffic controllers at the working position. She joined Airbus Group in 2006, as a human factor specialist for cockpit design and certification on different programs. She was in charge of the Cognitive Ergonomics Team in the Human Factors Department for several years. She moved to the R&T field, working on several topics including future cockpit design for Airbus Commercial but also road mapping in the Airbus Group. For several years, she has been contributing to the exploration of new capabilities and methods, especially eye-tracking technologies, to assess human performance in human factor evaluations.

Gilles Devreux (PhD) is a human factors specialist for the Human Design Group, now focused on neuro-ergonomics for Airbus Commercial. He has conducted research on human information behaviors and eye-tracking technologies in various fields such as road safety, the operating room, air traffic management, and aircraft cockpit design. He also participates in research in mixed reality with the BCOM Institute of Research and Technologies. He studied cognitive science at Lyon 2 Lumières University and psychology of learning at Paris Nanterre University. He obtained his PhD in psychology in 2015 from Toulouse Jean Jaures University /Champollion INU in Albi.

Eric Groen (PhD) is a senior scientist at Human Factors Department of Netherlands Organization for Applied Scientific Research (Nederlandse Organisatie voor Toegepast Natuurwetenschappelijk Onderzoek – TNO and a visiting professor at Cranfield University (UK). His research activities are aimed at improving simulator training for pilots to deal with non-normal conditions, such as airplane upsets, aerodynamic stall, or hypoxia. In the worst case, these conditions may lead to controlled flight into terrain (CFIT) or loss of control in flight (LOC-I). Eric has authored more than 100 scientific papers on topics involving: simulator motion cueing, human modeling, aerospace physiology, multimodal displays, spatial disorientation, motion sickness, upset prevention and recovery training (UPRT), startle and surprise management, and transfer of training.

Julia Harfmann is an accredited aviation psychologist with 5 years of experience in the application of human factors in the air traffic management sector. The main focus of her work is the identification and mitigation of key human error risks in major change programs through user-centered design, human factors training, and lessons learned from incident investigations. She also leads human factors work in various projects in the SESAR Horizon 2020 program. Julia gained her master's degree from the University of Graz, Austria, in 2016. Her research focused on the relationship between systematic debriefing and teamwork as well as their impact on safety culture in air traffic management. Julia is a member of the European Association for Aviation Psychology (EAAP).

Alexander Heintz graduated in clinical, instructional, and work/organizational psychology from the University of Heidelberg, Germany. He works as an ATM human factors expert at DFS Air Navigation Services Academy, mainly in the domain of selection and training of air traffic controllers and other operational roles in ATM. He has been involved in the human performance management activities of the European ATM Research and Development Program SESAR for more than 10 years. Alexander has been a member of various pan-European expert groups and of working arrangements in the EUROCONTROL and FAB framework around ATM human factors and training. His research focuses on the development and validation of psychological aptitude selection, human factors assurance activities, and cost–benefit analysis for human factors and training in aviation.

Mauro Marchitto (PhD) graduated in psychology (University of Padua, Italy) in 2004. After a thesis prepared at the Joint Research Center of the European Commission (Ispra, Italy), he worked in a private company as a human factors trainer in aviation maintenance and as researcher on several European projects. He moved to the University of Granada (Spain) in 2008, obtaining an MSc in cognitive neuroscience (2009), working in the Cognitive Ergonomics Group, and finally obtaining a PhD in social sciences (2015), with a thesis on the application of eye-tracking technologies to measure cognitive complexity in air traffic control. He moved to Paris for postdoctoral studies in 2015 (LUTIN Lab, University Paris VIII), working on methodologies for cognitive workload measurement. He joined Airbus (Toulouse) in 2019, as a human factors specialist, in the R&T domain for future cockpit design, in particular focusing on multidimensional assessment in human factors evaluations.

Renée Pelchen-Medwed is a human factors expert with almost 20 years of experience in the aviation industry. She has a master's degree in psychology from the Karl Franzens University in Graz, Austria. She joined EURO-CONTROL in 2003. In the past 10 years she worked mainly in the Single European Sky ATM Research (SESAR) program. In SESAR 1 she contributed to the development of the human performance assessment process for SESAR and was then responsible for leading and performing human performance assessments in various operational and technical SESAR projects. Recently, Renée was seconded to EASA as an air traffic management expert working on different HF and safety-related topics in the ATM domain.

Florence Reuzeau is an aeronautical engineer and doctor in cognitive ergonomics. She worked as a safety specialist on complex avionics systems for 5 years before setting up the Human Factors Organization in Airbus Engineering. She integrated human sciences into engineering for an optimized human-centered design applied to A380, A400M, A350, and ATR aircraft. She contributed to the definition of human factors regulations. Since 2014, she has been the human factors executive expert for Airbus overall, defining the Airbus Group human factors strategy for research and development. She is involved in international standardization groups and very active in the organization of human factors conferences worldwide. She is a European expert for European project evaluation.

Luca Save is a human factors and safety expert, with 20 years of experience in safety-critical systems and a special interest in aviation and railway transport. In 2003 he received his PhD degree in cognitive ergonomics, with a scholarship funded by the Italian National Railway Company. For 9 years he has been a lecturer in human–machine interaction at the University of Siena. Since 2005 he has worked as consultant and R&D manager for the Italian company Deep Blue srl, where he specializes in the air traffic management domain. In the context of the SESAR Program, he has been coordinating a project dealing with the development of guidelines for human performance automation support.

Michaela Schwarz (PhD) is an accredited aviation psychologist and human factors expert working toward improving human performance in aviation and rail. She received her doctoral degree in psychology from the University of Graz, Austria, in 2016. Her main research focus and expertise is the assessment and improvement of safety and just culture, the integration of human performance elements in safety management systems, and the development and delivery of human factors training programs. Michaela looks back on more than 15 years of experience working with aviation-related personnel including pilots, air traffic controllers, safety experts, accident investigators, and authorities. Michaela is President of the European Association for Aviation Psychology (EAAP) and Vice-Chair of the Austrian Aviation Psychology Association.

Christiane Uhlig is a specialist for quality assurance in health care. She is responsible for the external quality report in the Märkische Kliniken Holding, Lüdenscheid. In addition, she works as a psychologist in several projects dedicated to prevention and health psychology. She is involved in nursing education at various nursing chapels in Germany. In particular she looks at evidence-based nursing. As a pain nurse, she is responsible for the acute pain department at the Klinikum Lüdenscheid, Germany. She received a doctoral degree in psychology by studying aspects of patient satisfaction in health-care services.

Thomas Uhlig is a psychologist and anesthetist. During the past 30 years he has conducted several studies on perioperative stress reactions. He has initiated several projects in health psychology dedicated to the impact of sports and exercise on aspects of health. In his clinical research in psychology, he focused on cognitive impairment after surgery and intensive care. In intensive care medicine his main emphasis lies on aspects of tissue oxygenation. He is an academic teacher in human factors and human resource management. He is Head of the Department of Anesthesiology and Intensive Care Medicine at the Klinikum Lüdenscheid in Germany.

Peer Commentaries

Methods in a broad sense are essential to both research and practice. This book offers a comprehensive overview essential to everyone in aviation and is an excellent tool box for both practitioners and researchers in aviation. Its comprehensive and future-oriented outlook on methods and techniques in aviation make it a unique contribution to the field of aviation psychology – a must for both researchers and practitioners.

Professor Monica Martinussen, PhD, Faculty of Health Sciences, UiT The Arctic University, Tromsø, Norway

This book takes a practitioner's approach to aviation psychology and provides an excellent, concisely written overview on important techniques and methods, including the current state of the art regarding the most frequently used psychophysiological measurements. All chapters are supplemented by a wealth of references for further reading. I particularly liked Eric Groen's brilliant overview on Spatial Disorientation Research, and obtained several interesting new insights on the biophysiology underlying stress and stress recovery from the chapter written by Thomas and Christiane Uhlig.

I am convinced that much of the material presented in this book is also highly relevant for people working in other fields of applied psychology, such as the automotive industry.

Christoph Vernaleken, DEng, Expert Human Factors Engineering, Airbus Defense & Space GmbH, Manching, Germany

The book reflects the evolution of the field of aviation psychology and human factors and presents many examples of contemporary research that contribute to enhancing aviation safety.

The book highlights the critical role of aviation psychology research in ensuring our advances in technology anticipate human factors issues and fully integrate a human factors perspective into new technologies across all aspects of aviation, from the flight deck to air traffic control, engineering, maintenance and beyond. The real strength of this book is the focus on bringing together aviation psychology with physiology. With chapters dedicated to the objective measurement of human performance including eye-tracking, cardiac, and other forms of physiological monitoring the book sets out an agenda for future research with an integrated and holistic perspective of contemporary human factors.

Matthew Thomas, PhD, Westwood-Thomas Associates and Central Queensland University, Australia